NEVADA THORNTON
Christmas

LARGE PRINT

Coloring books for adults relaxation

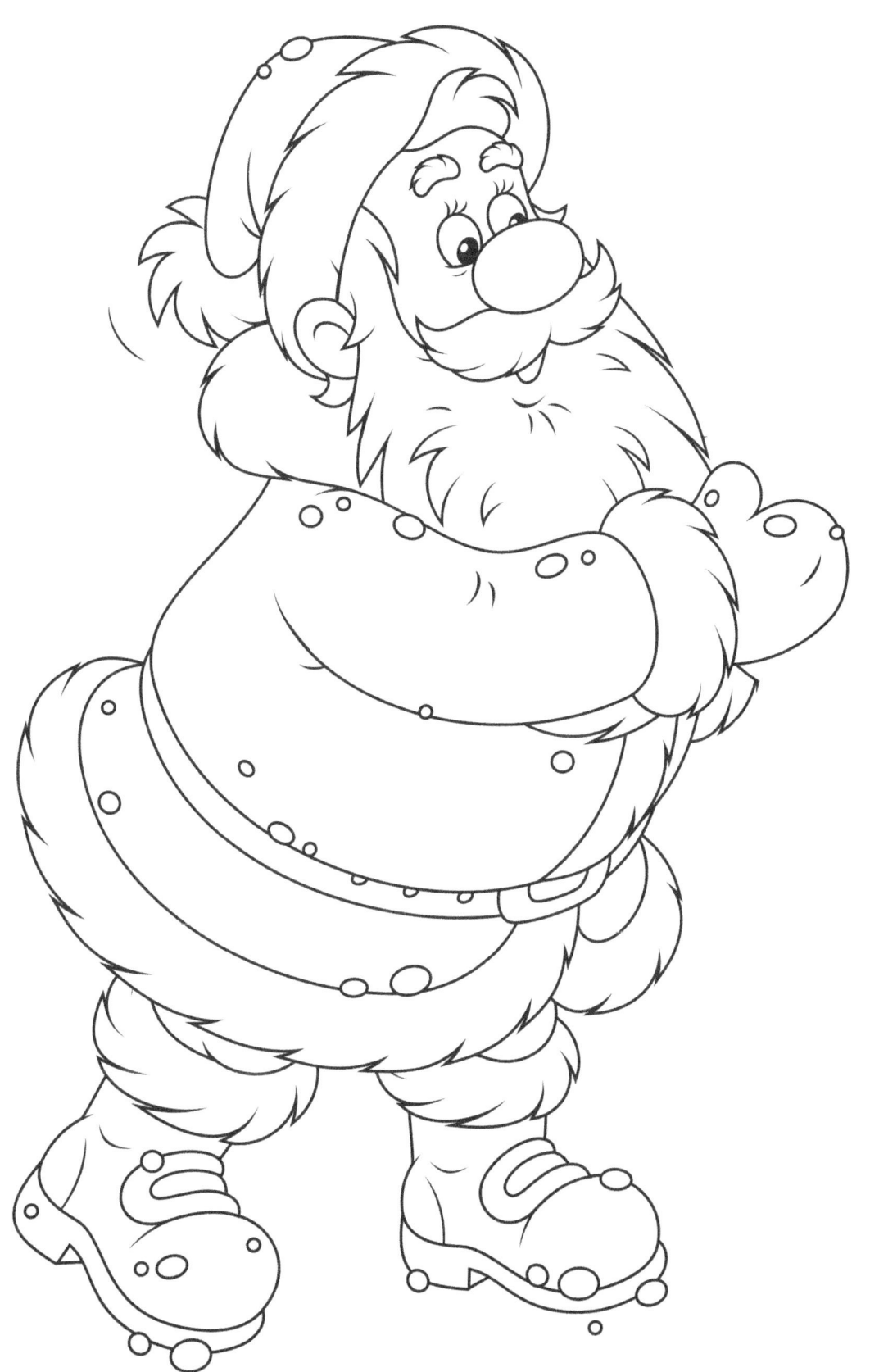

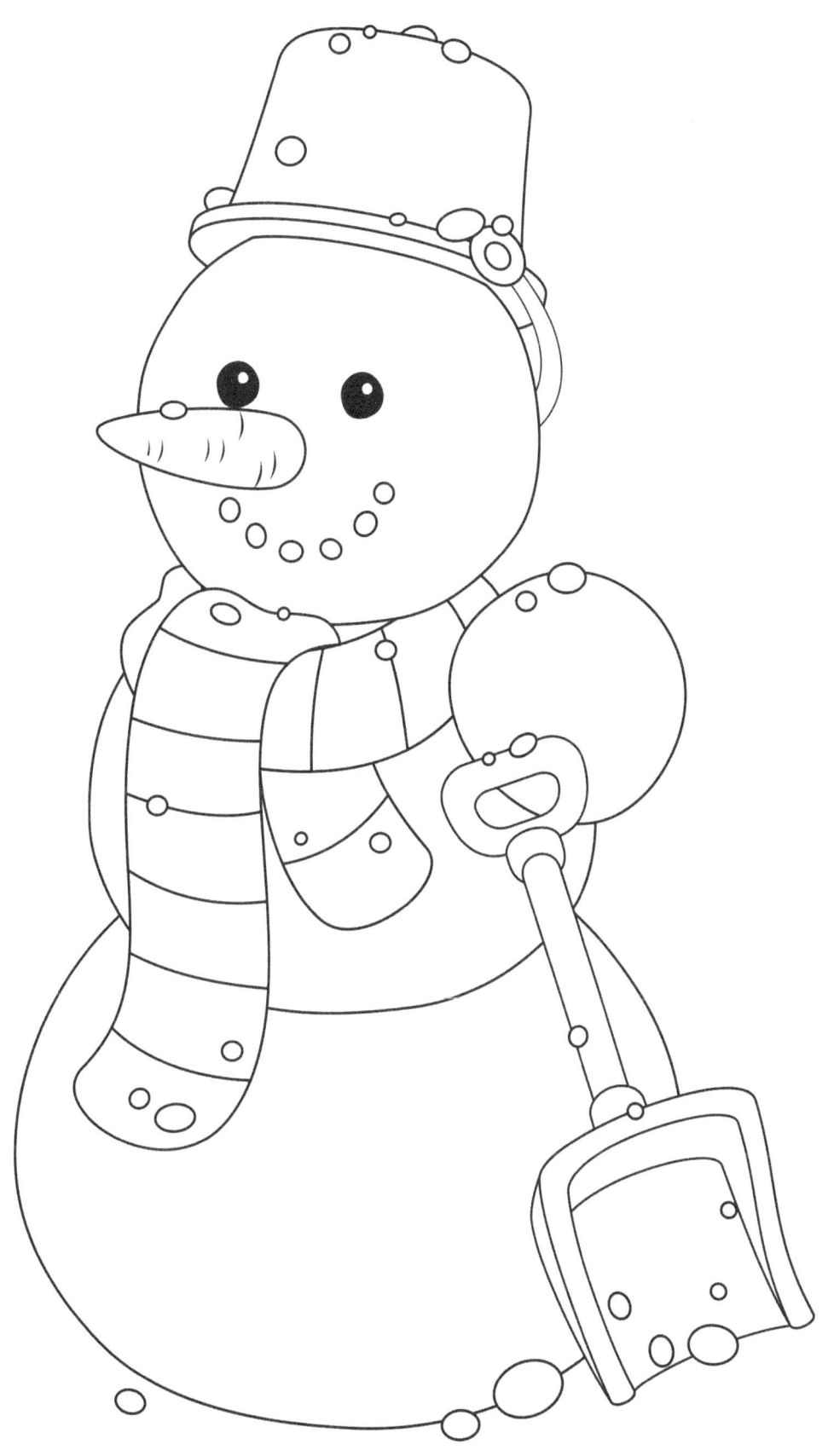

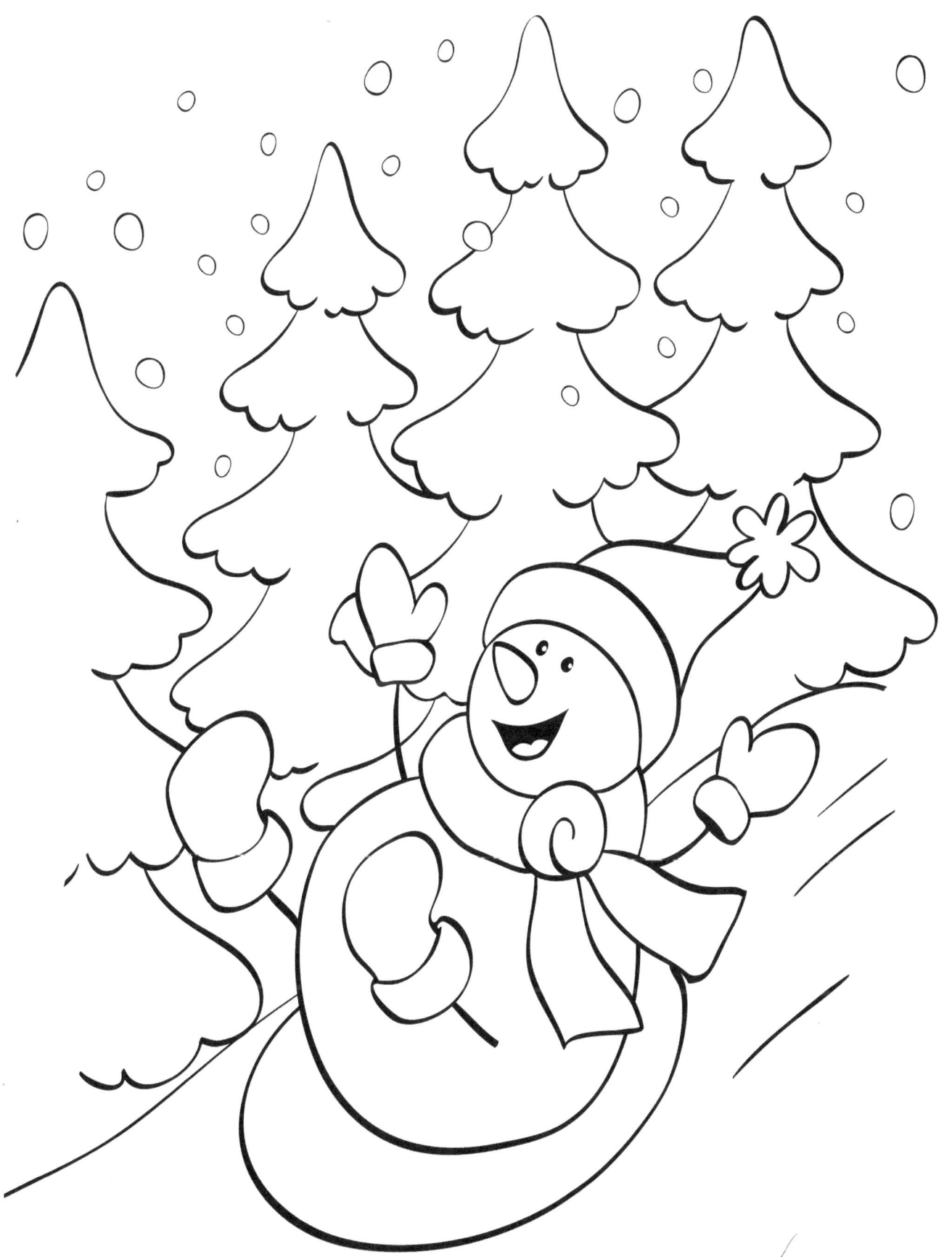

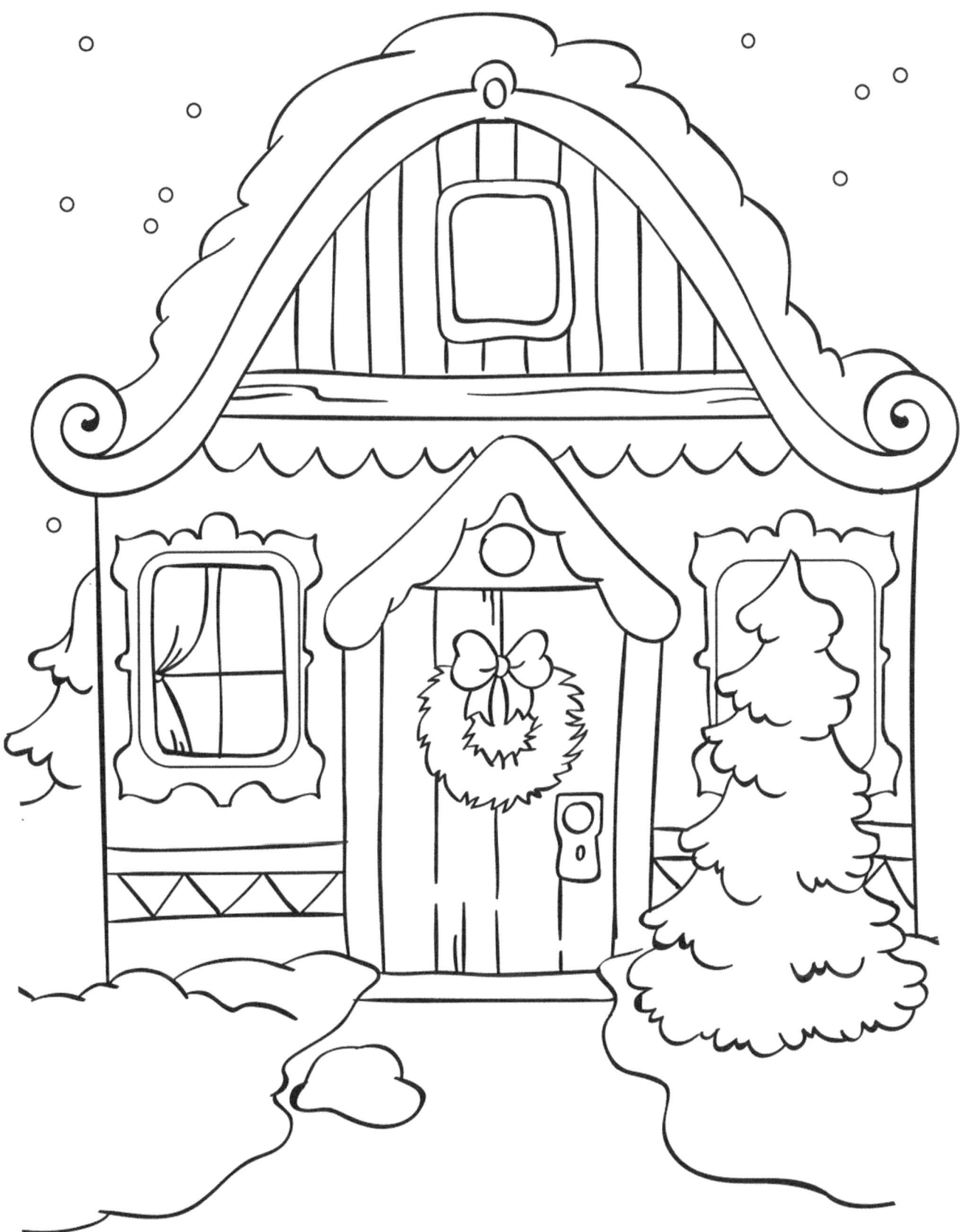

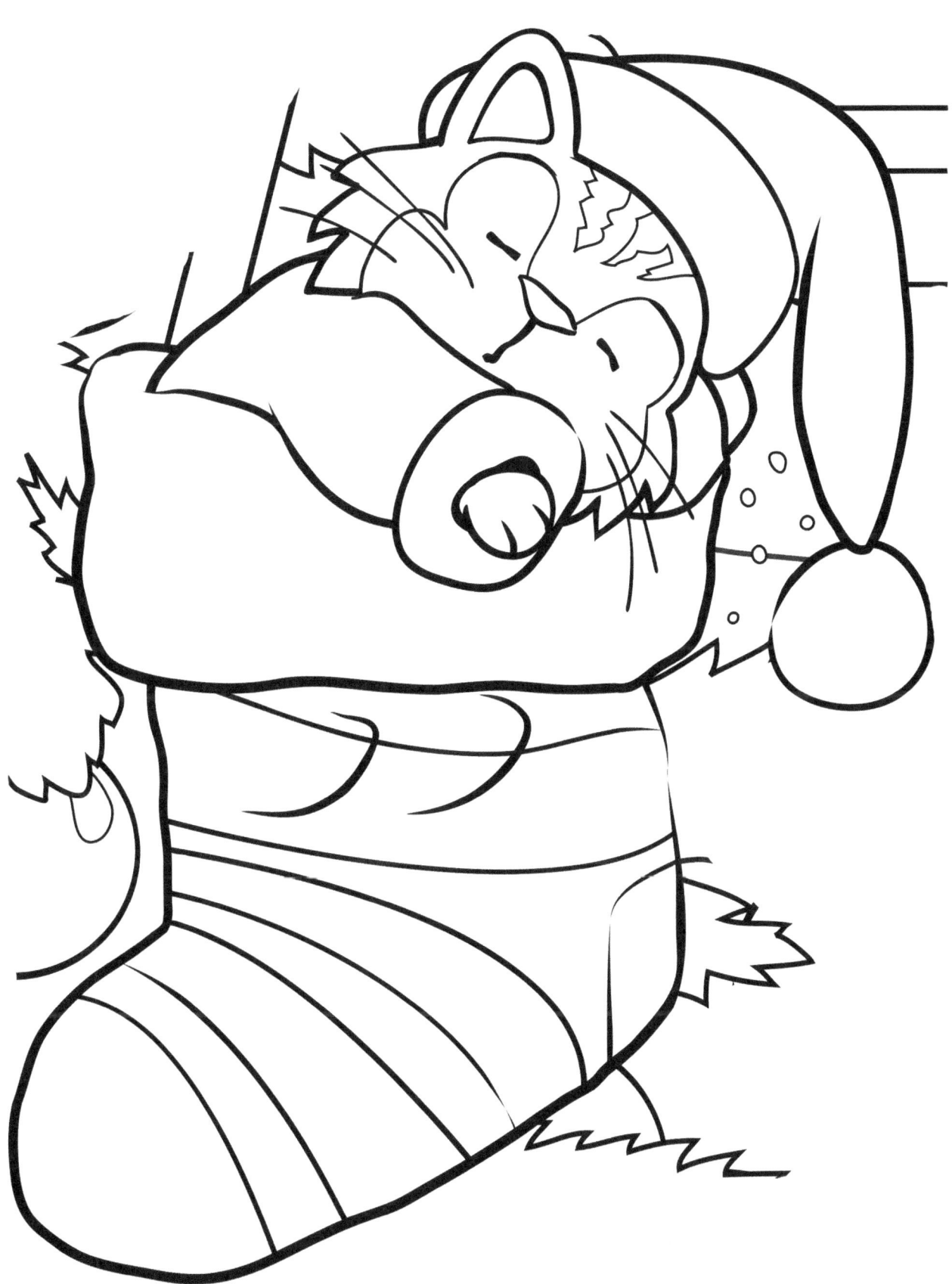

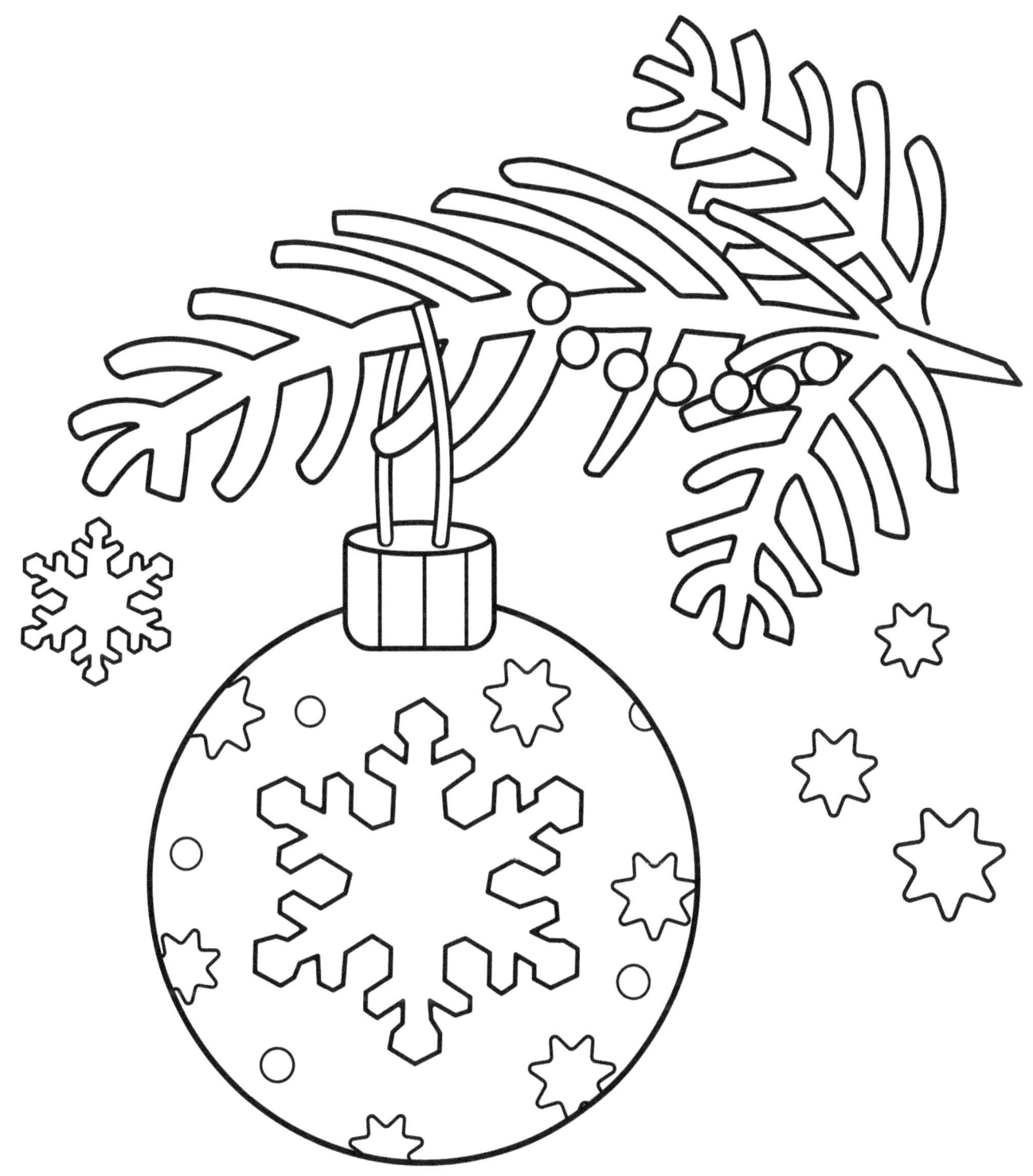

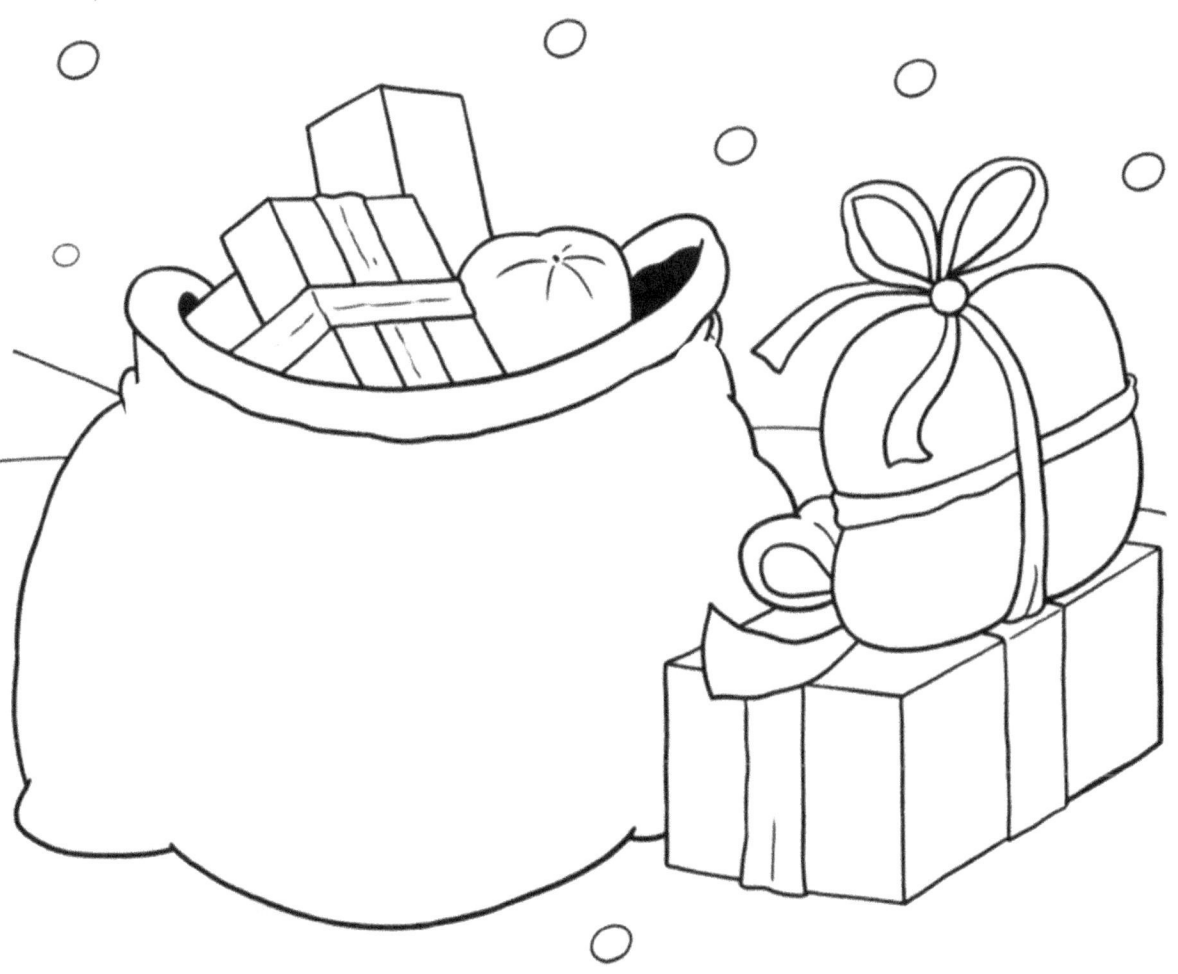

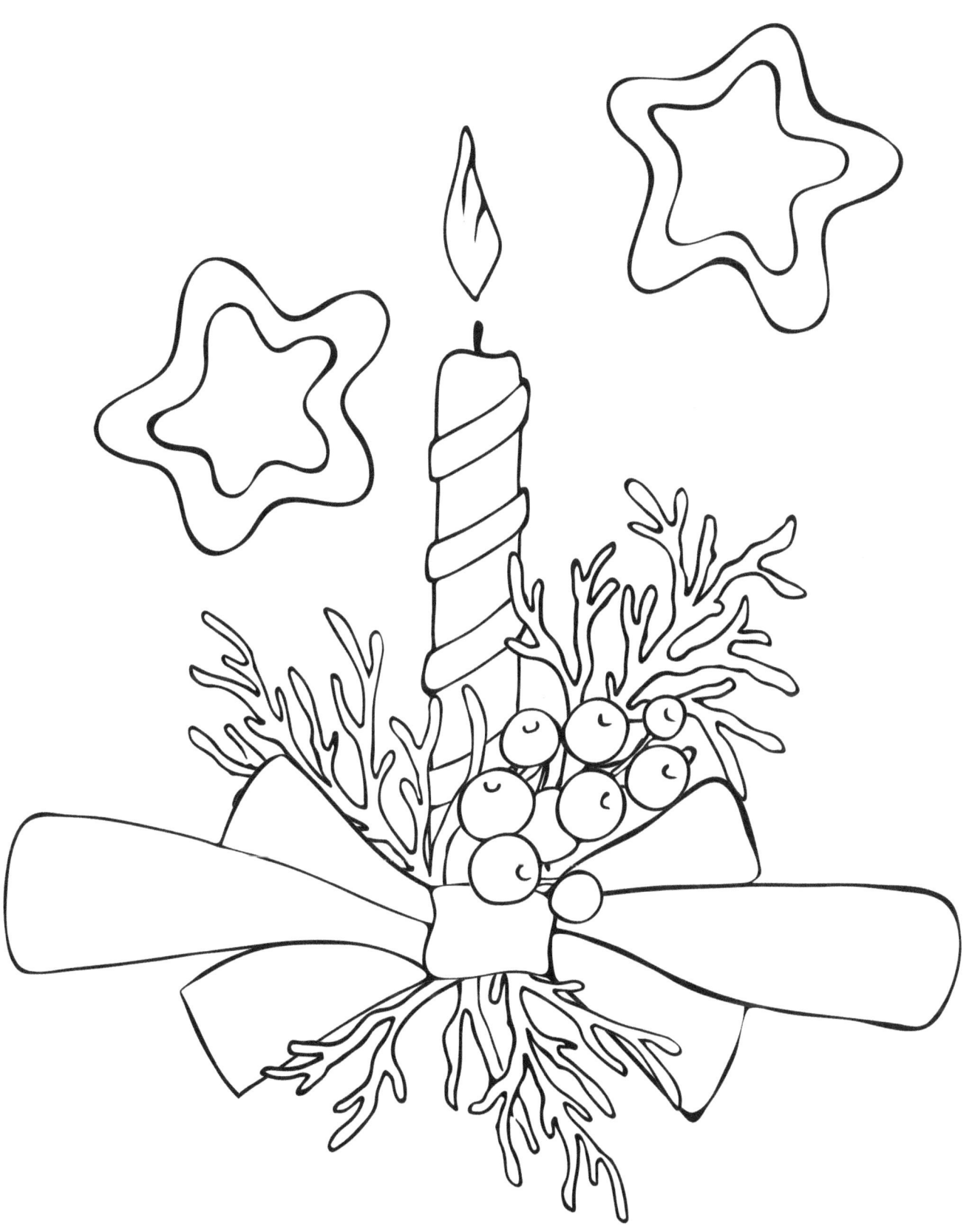

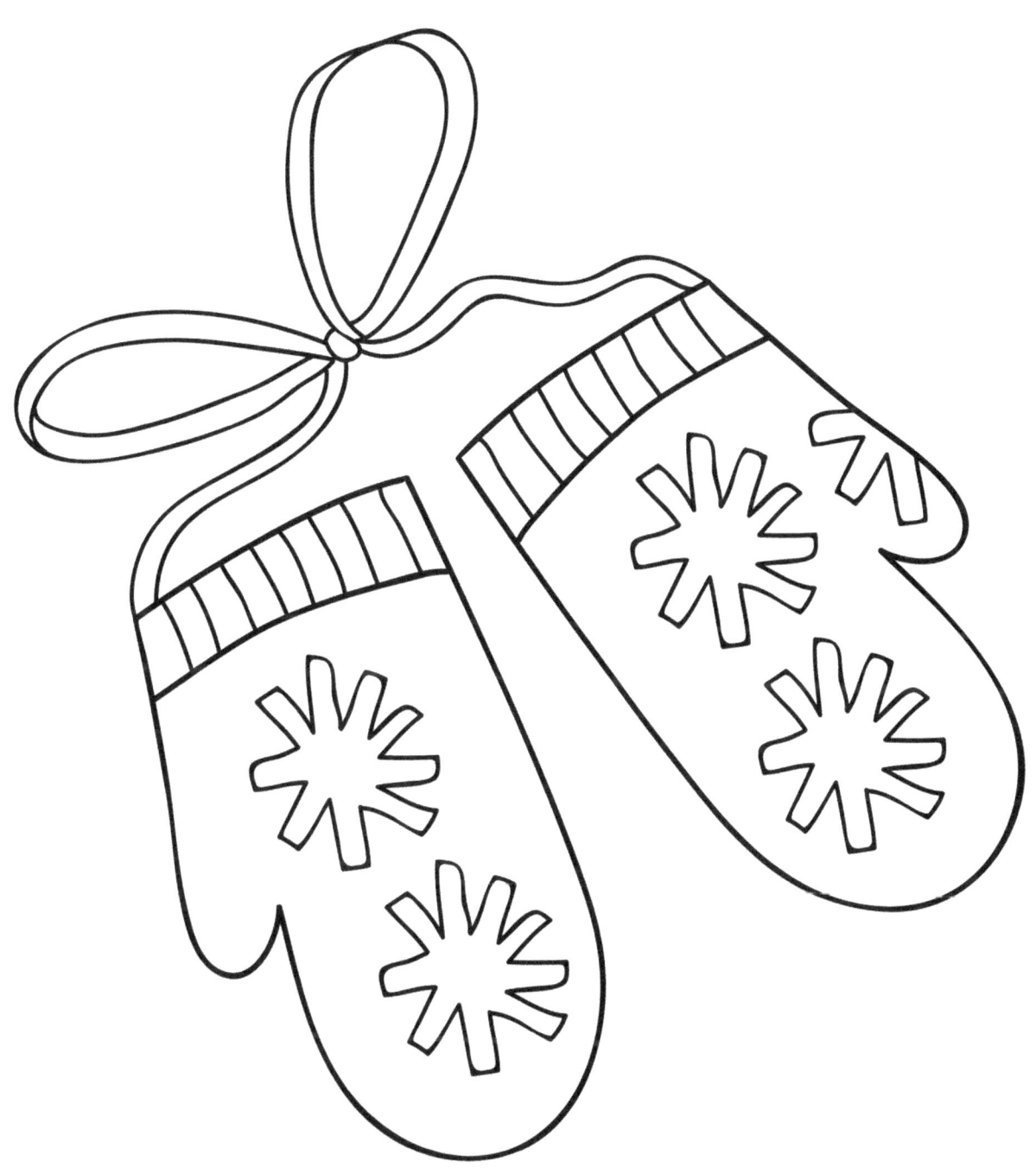

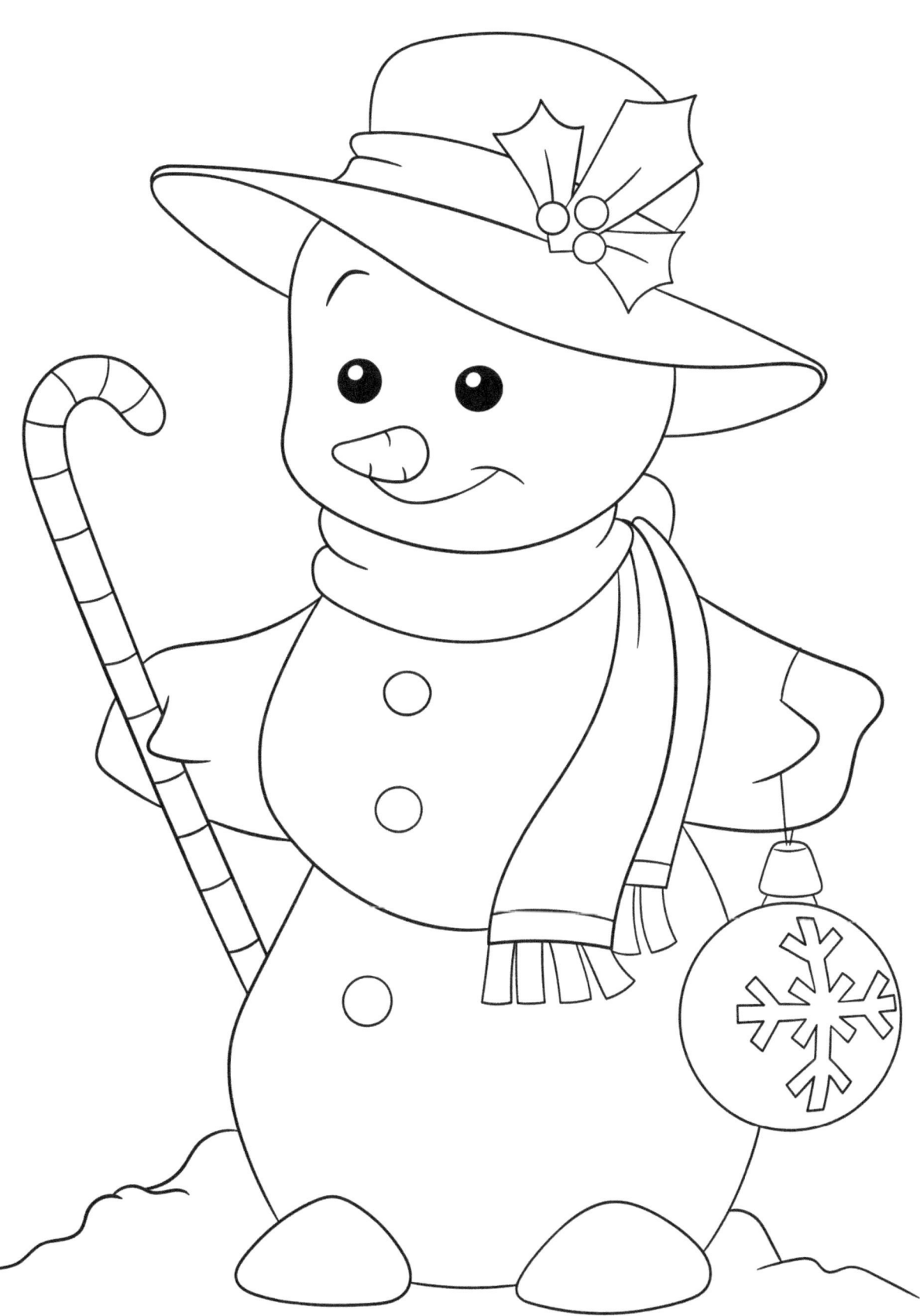

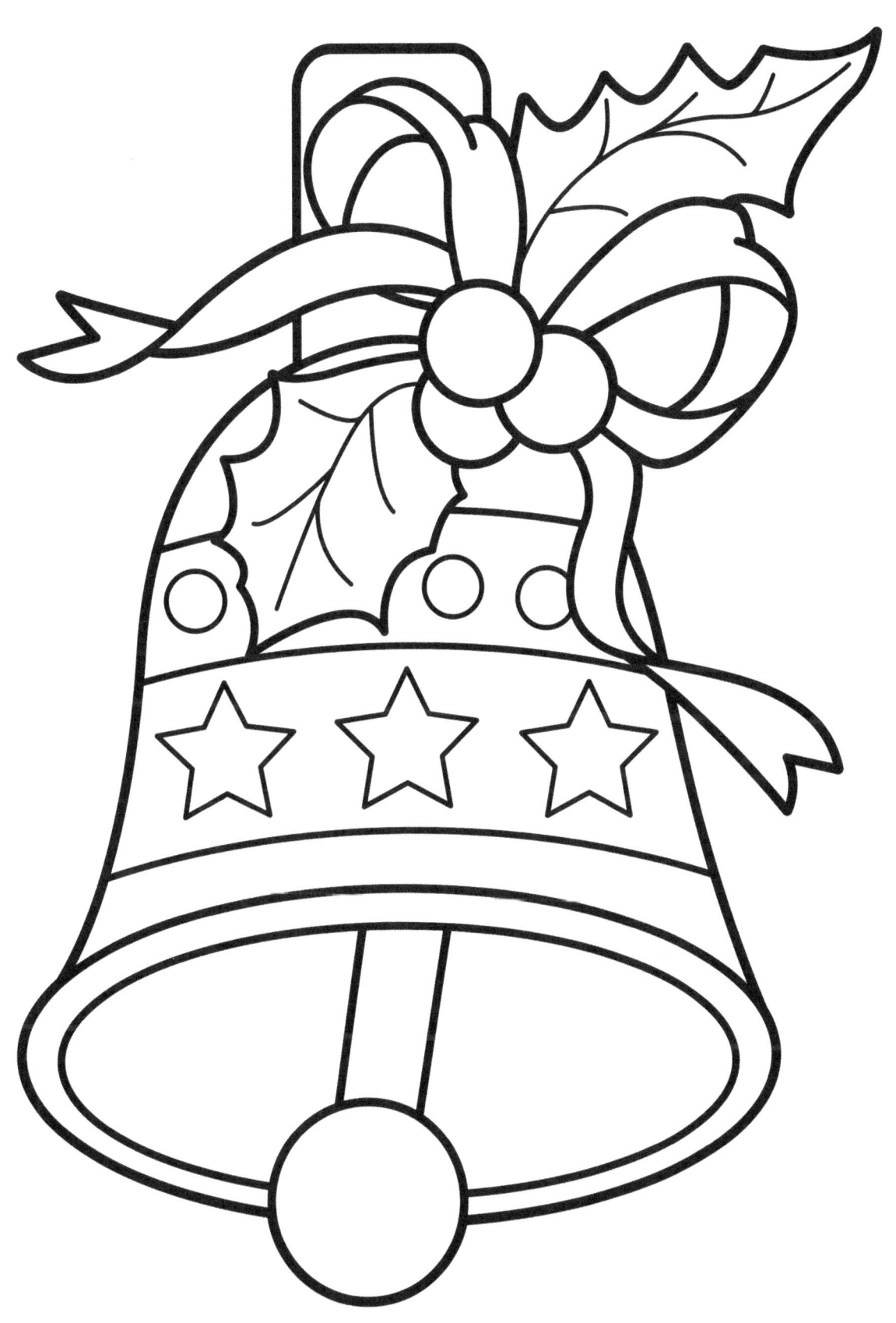

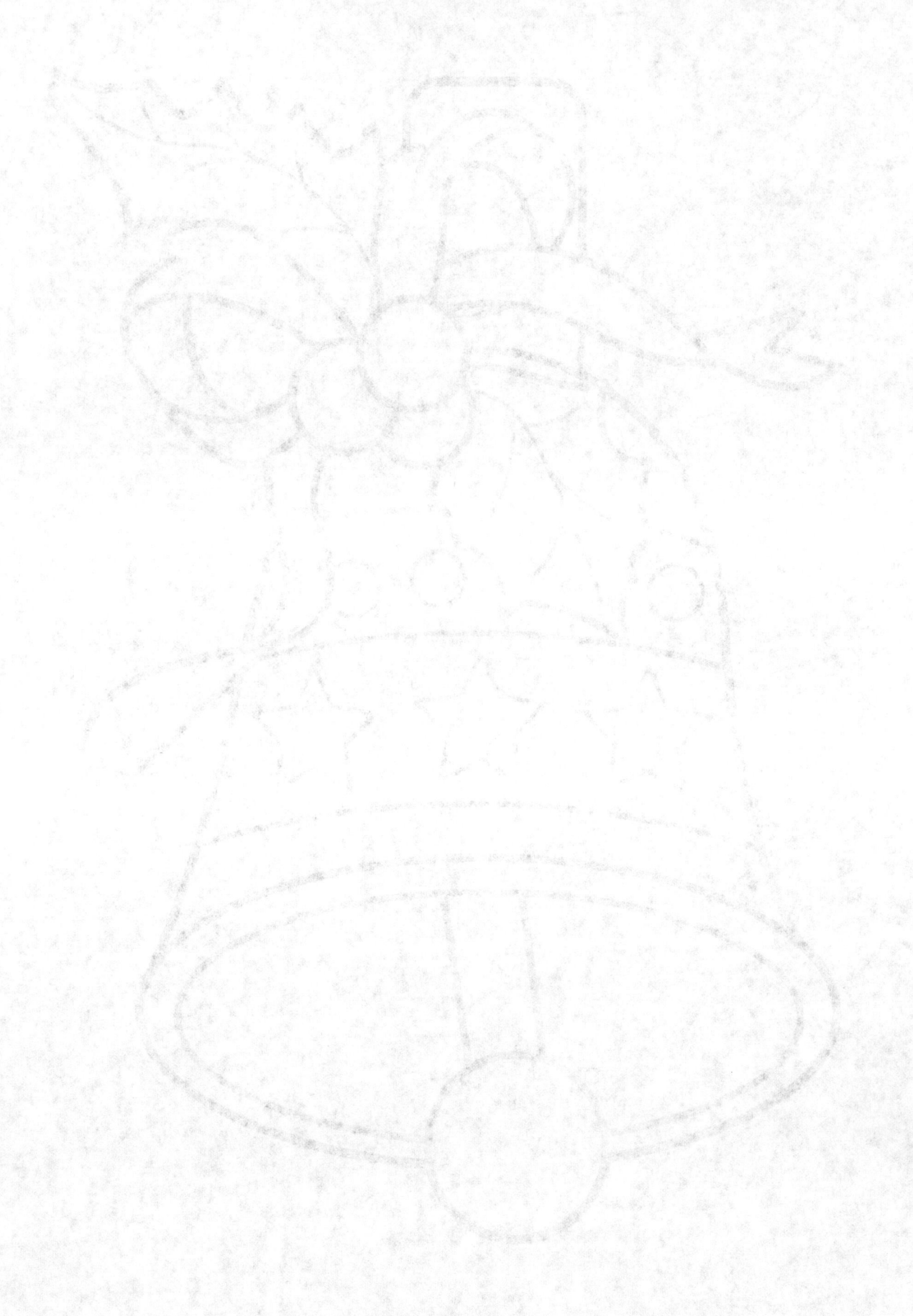

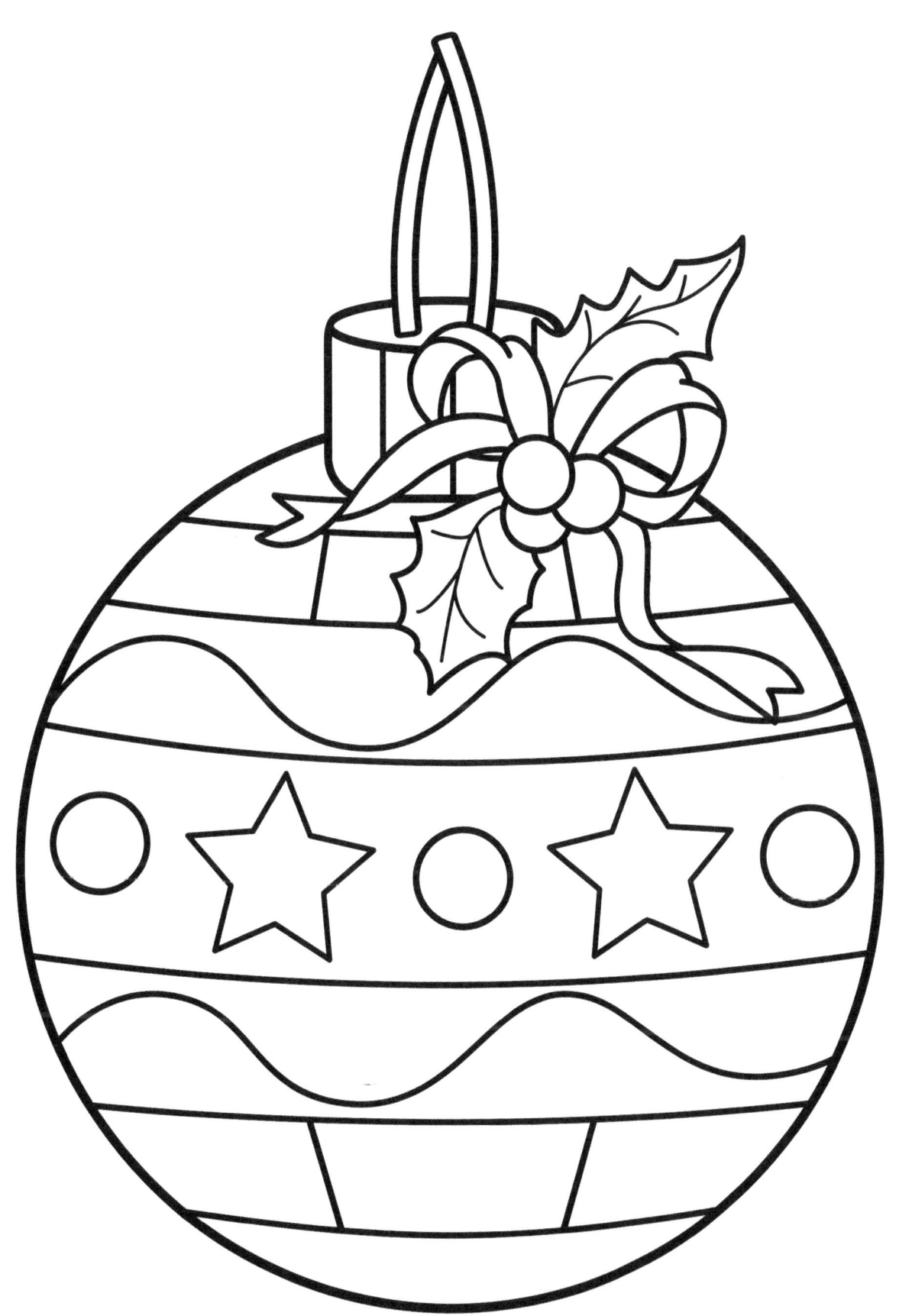

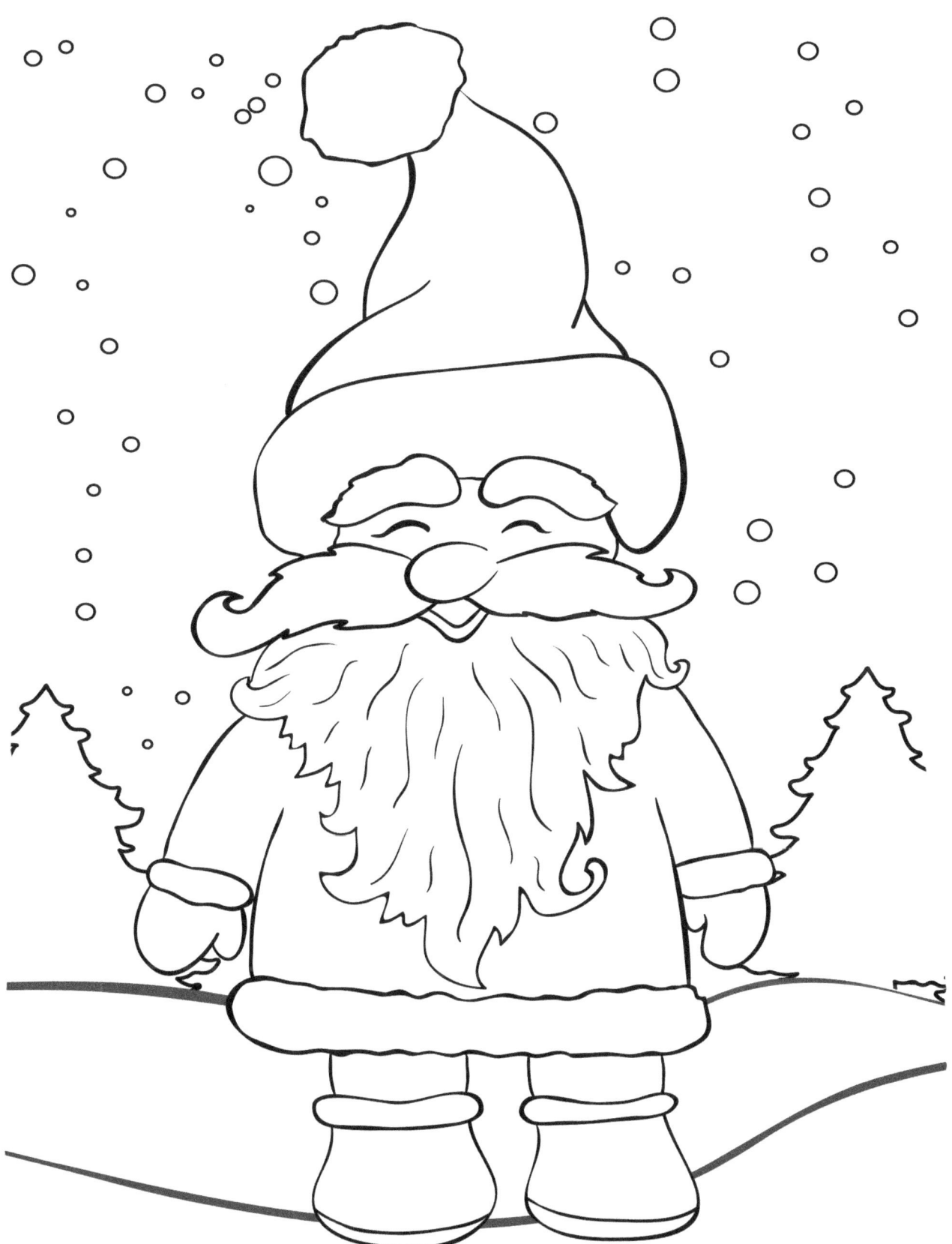

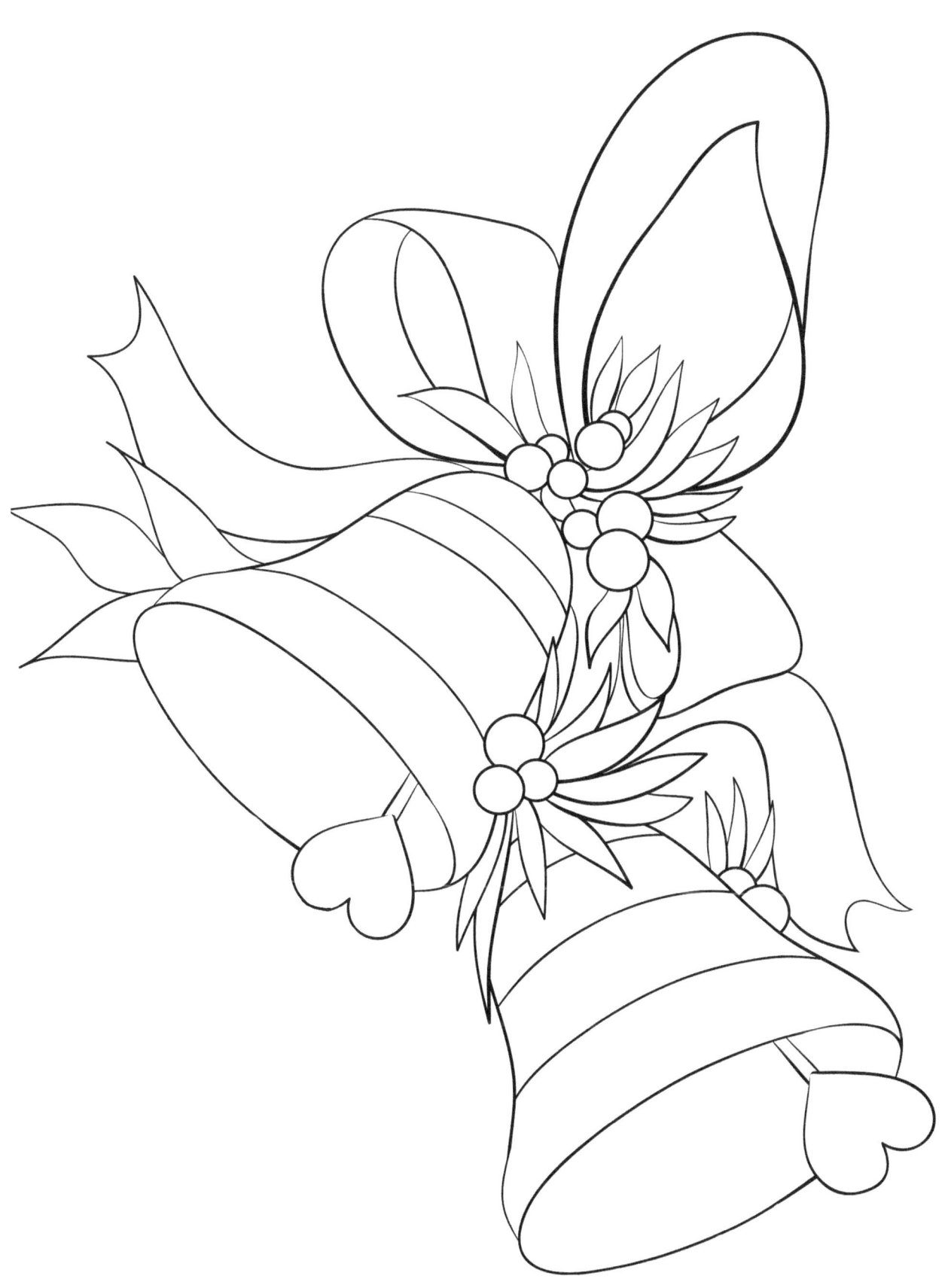

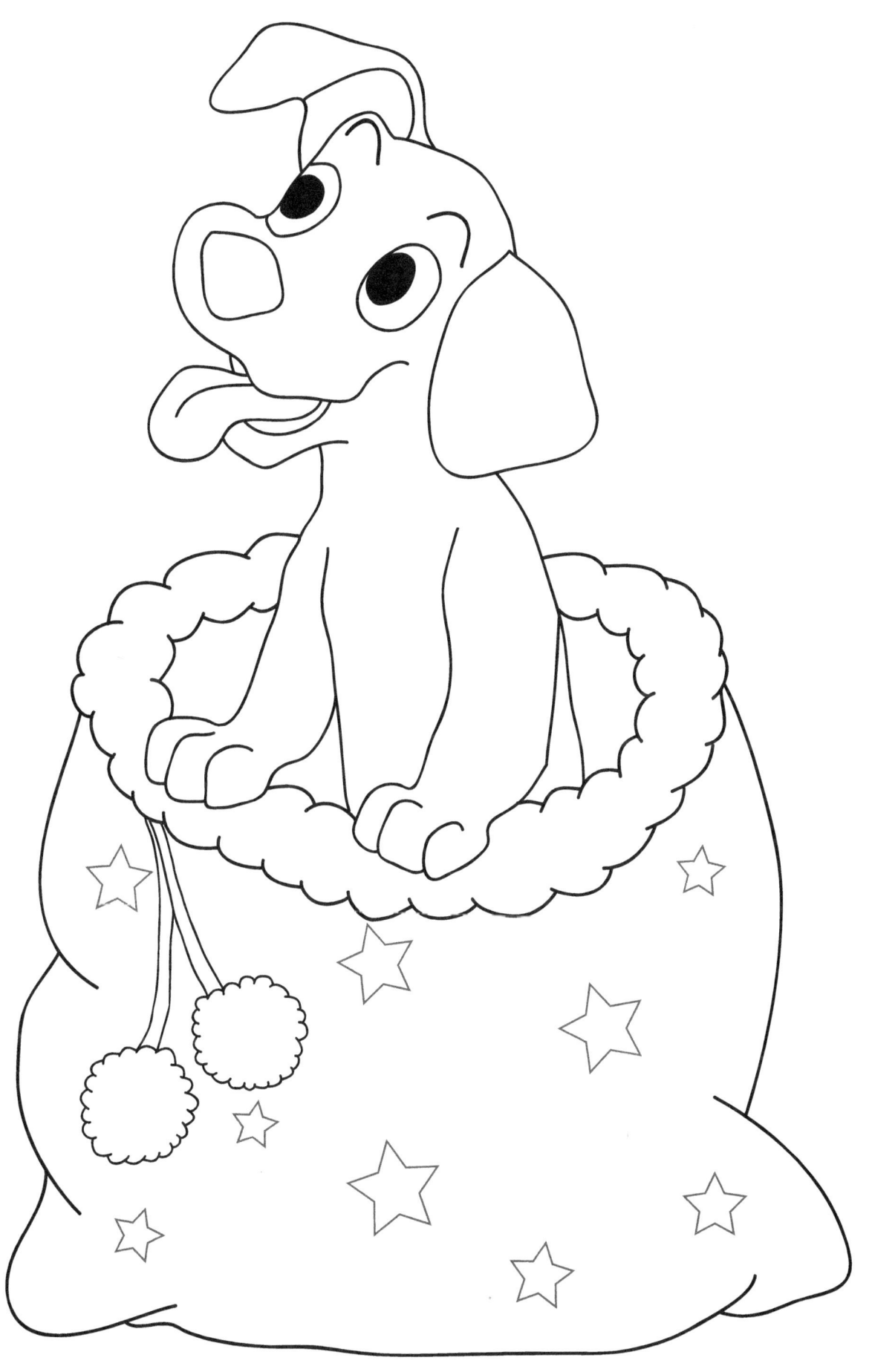

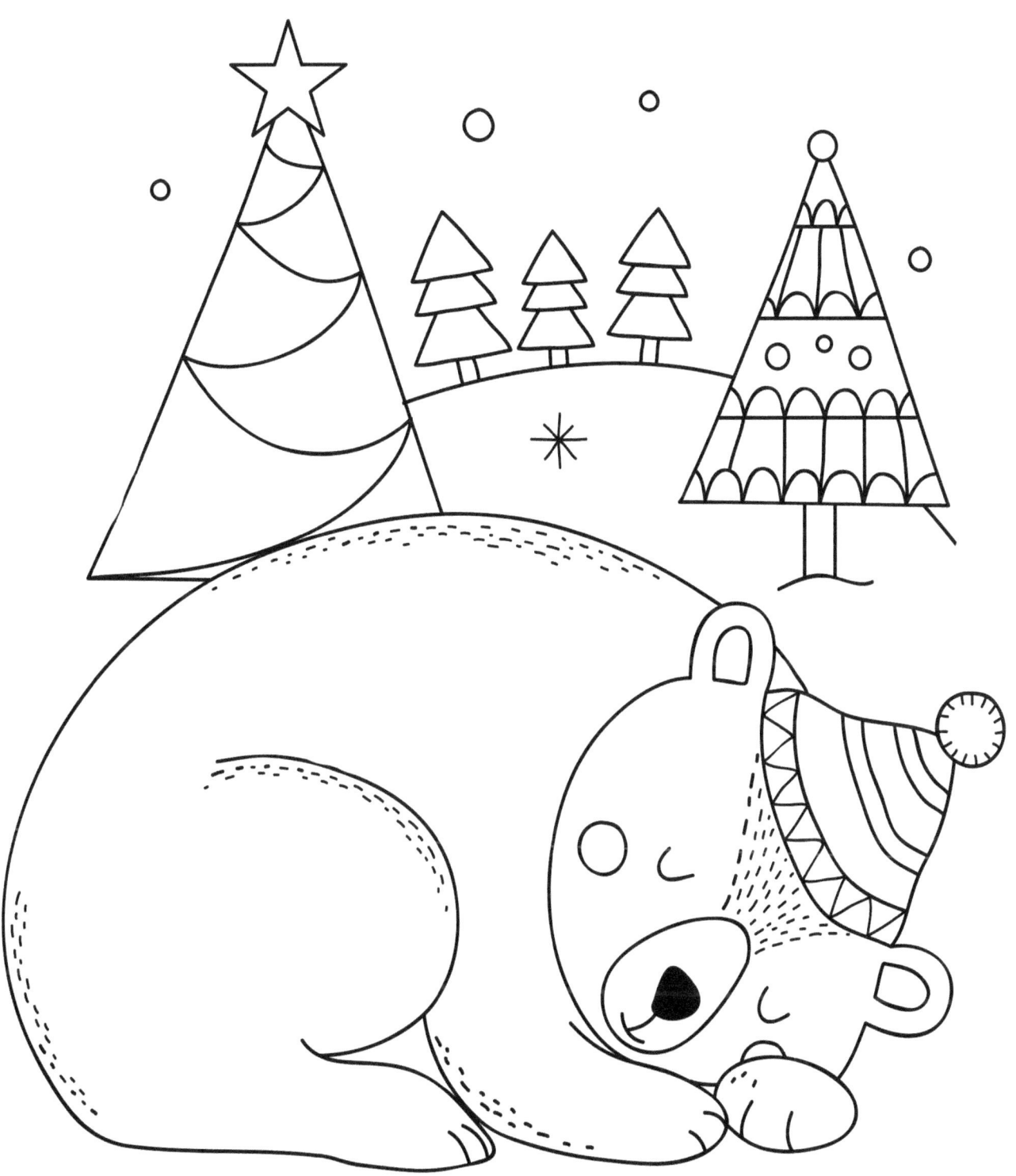

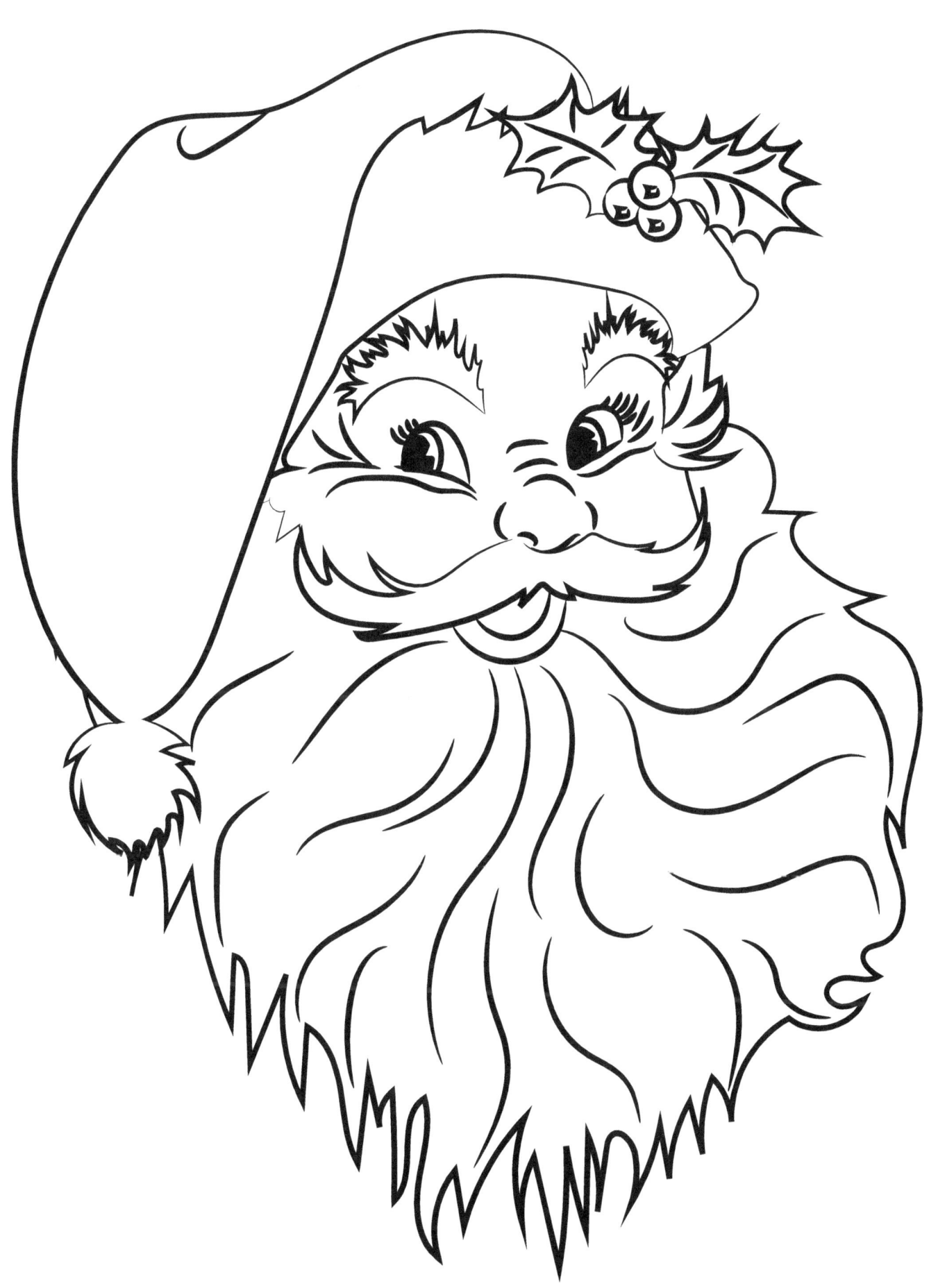

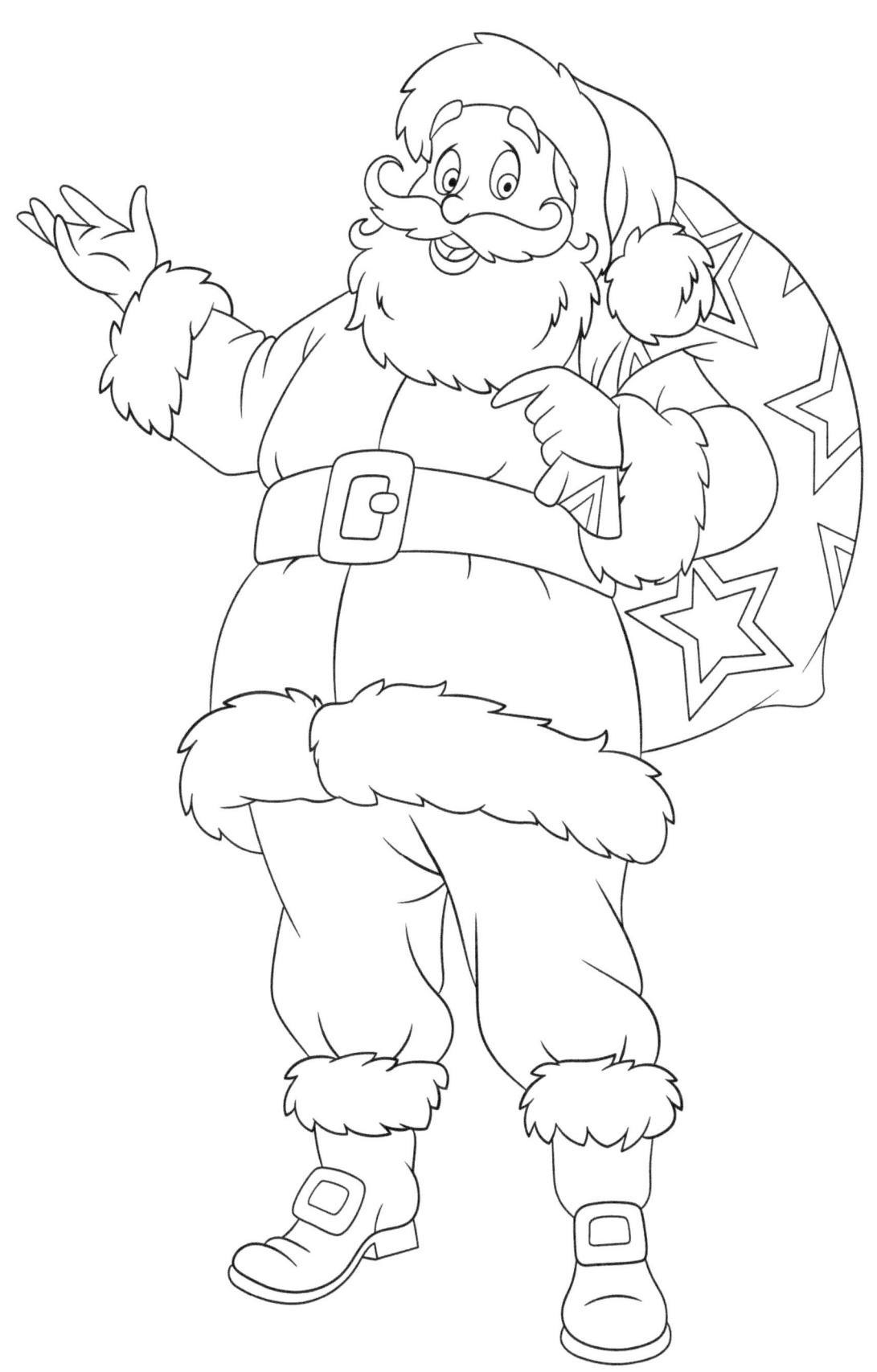

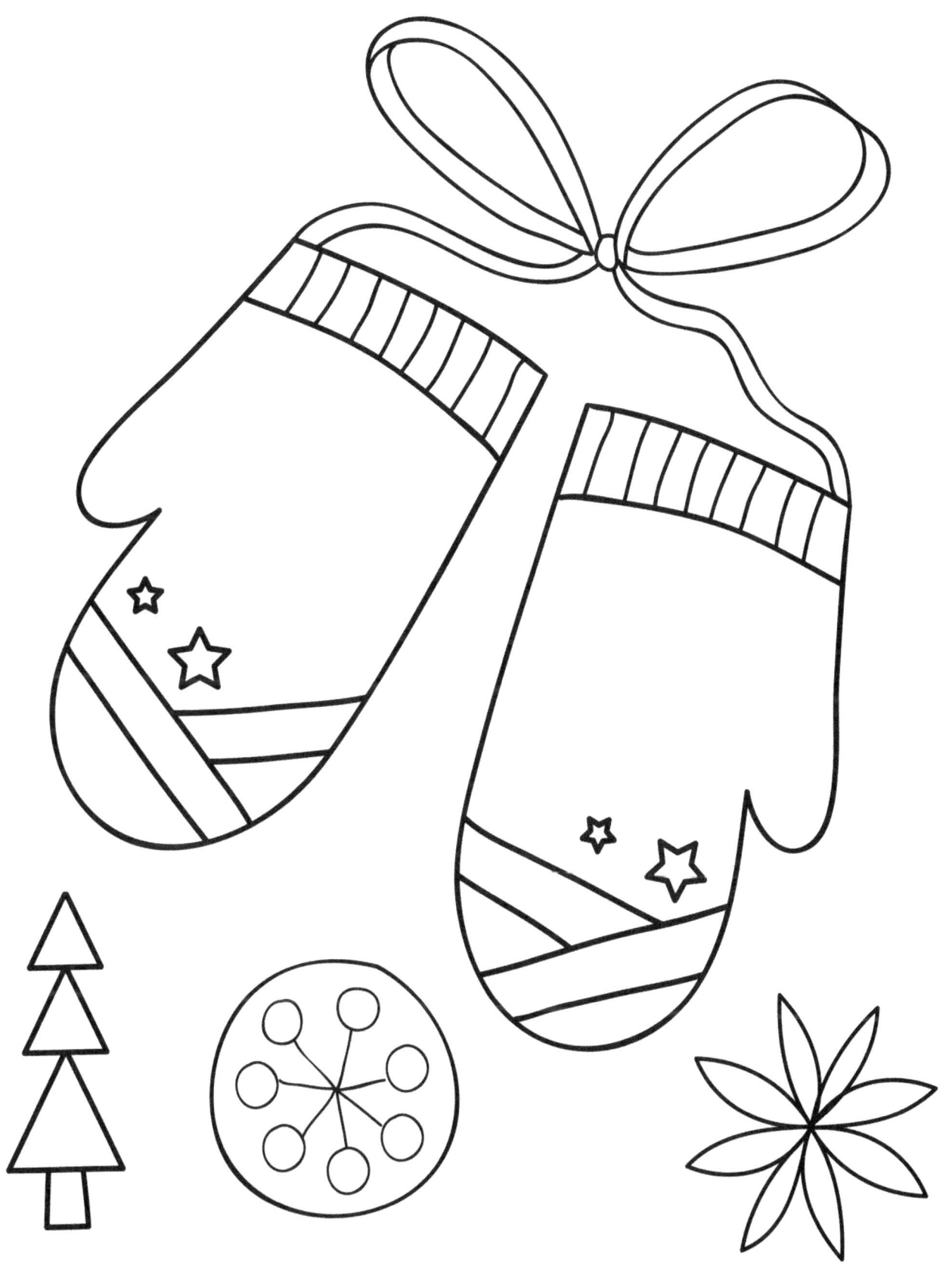

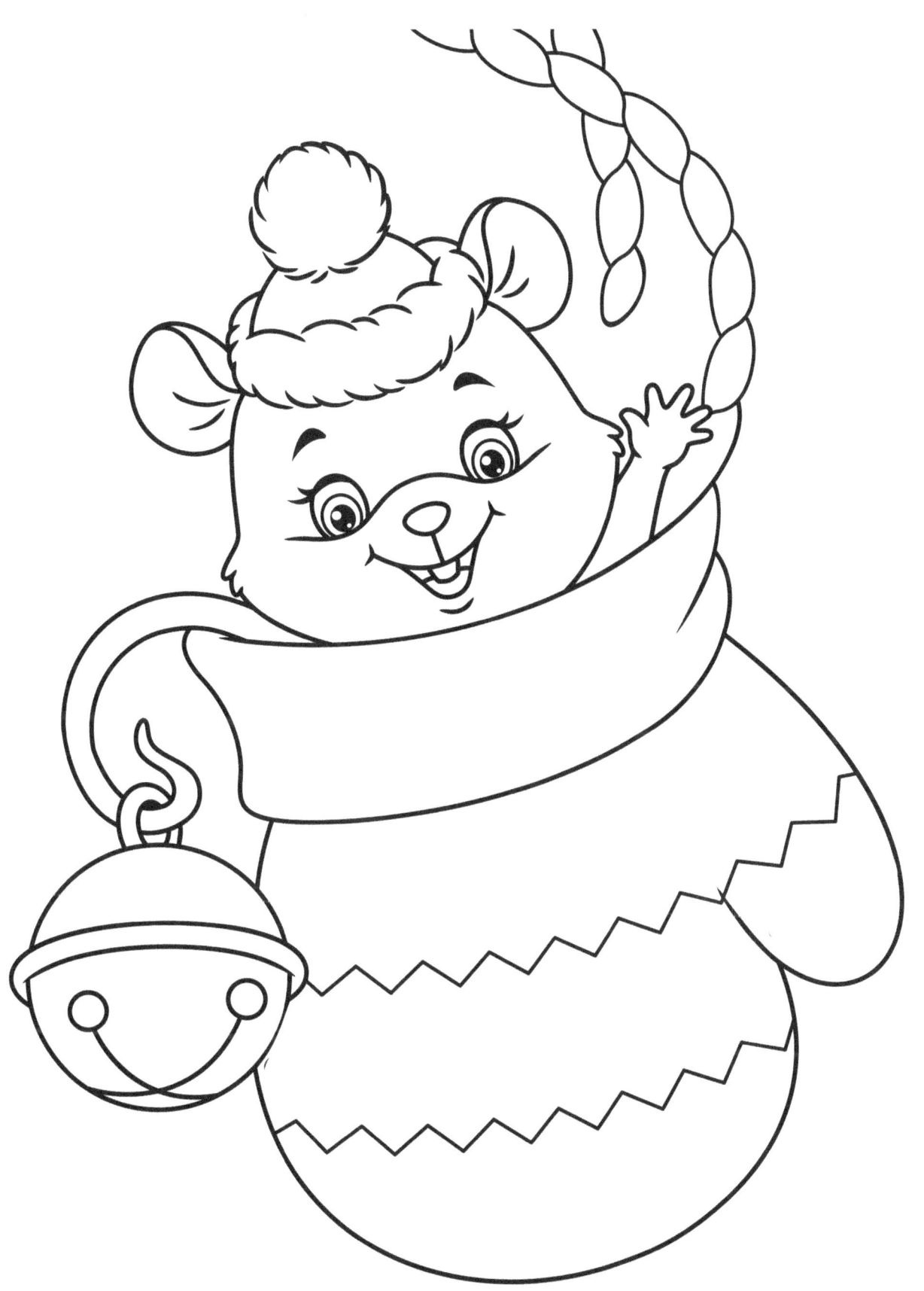

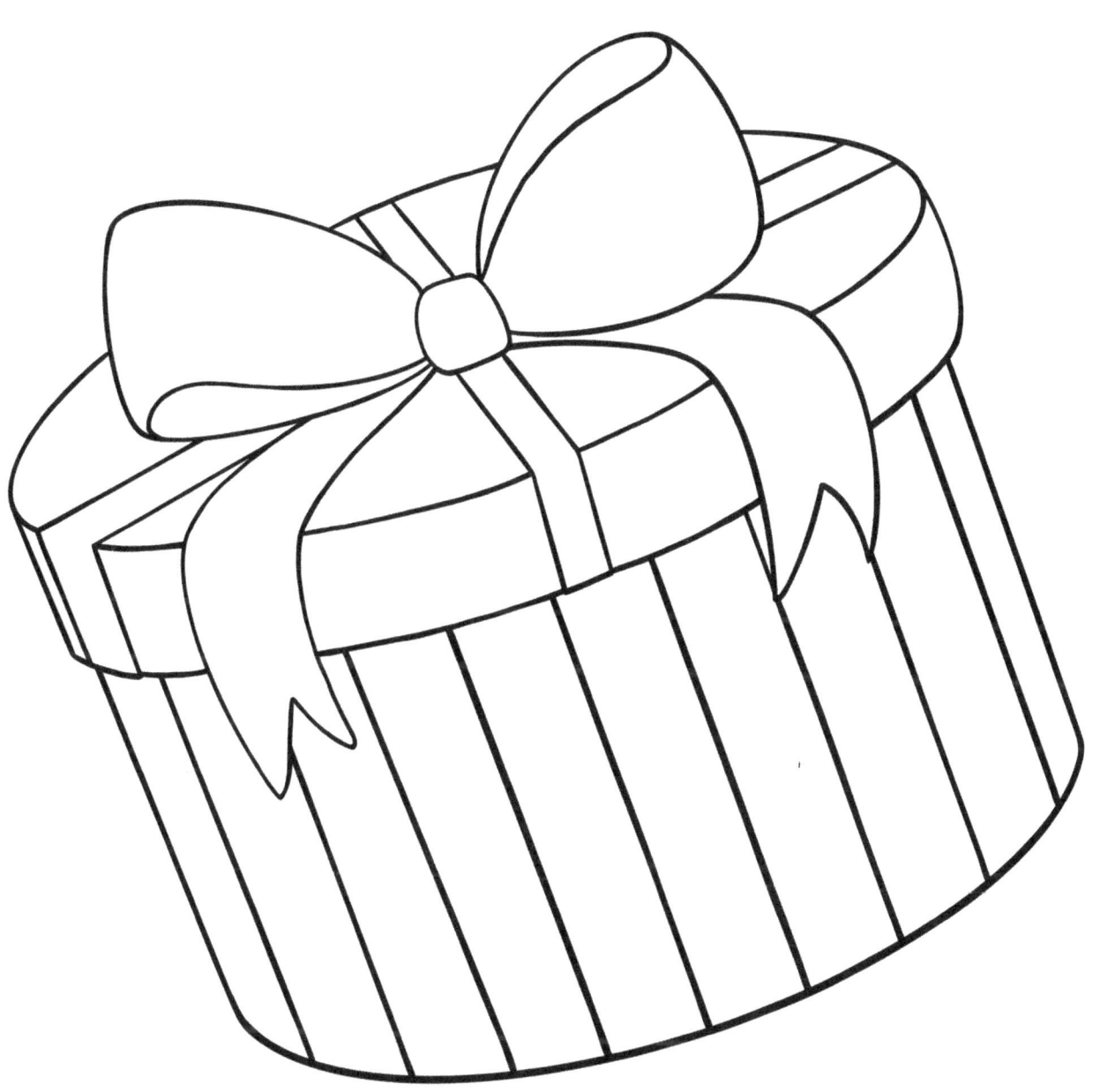

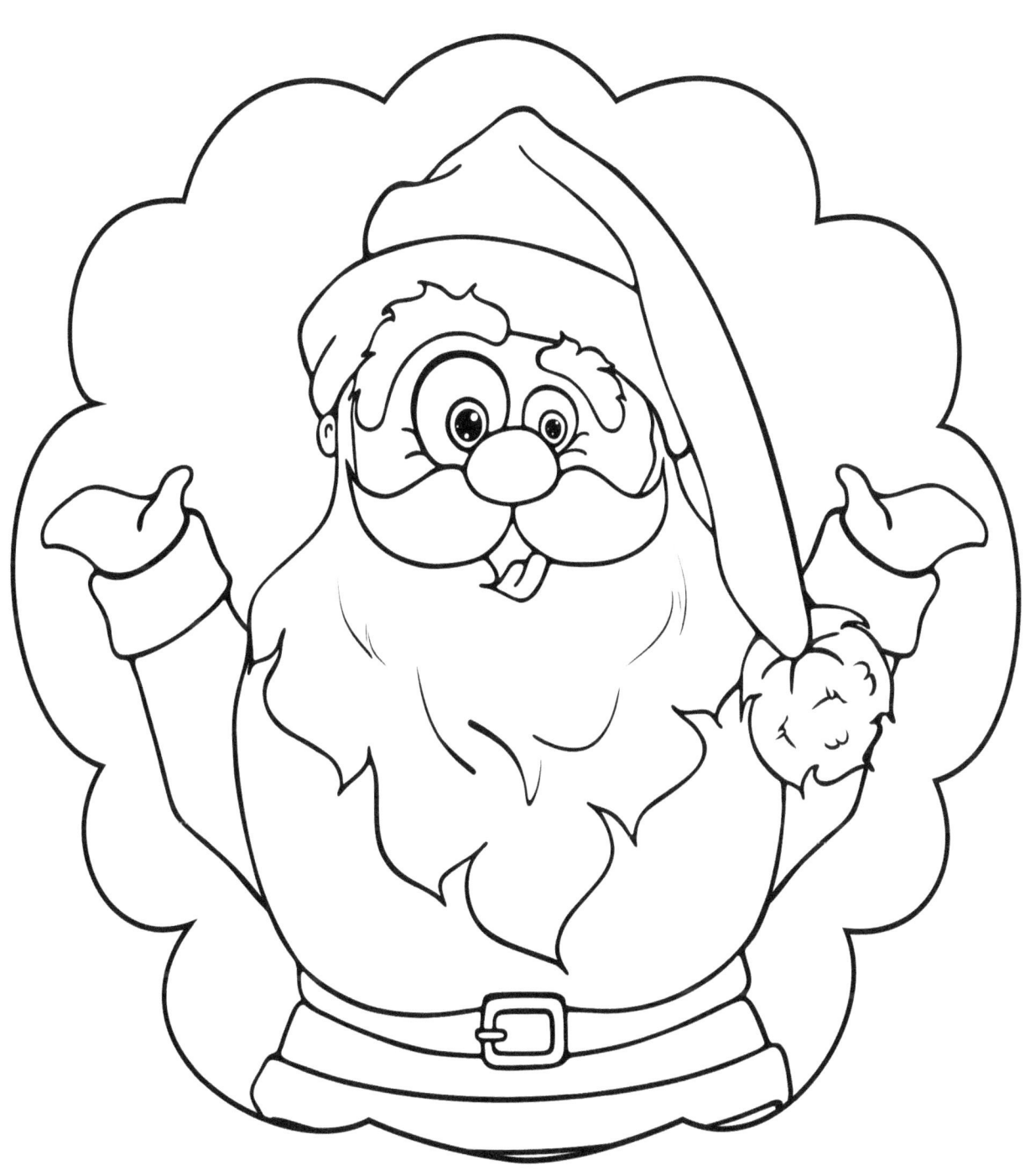

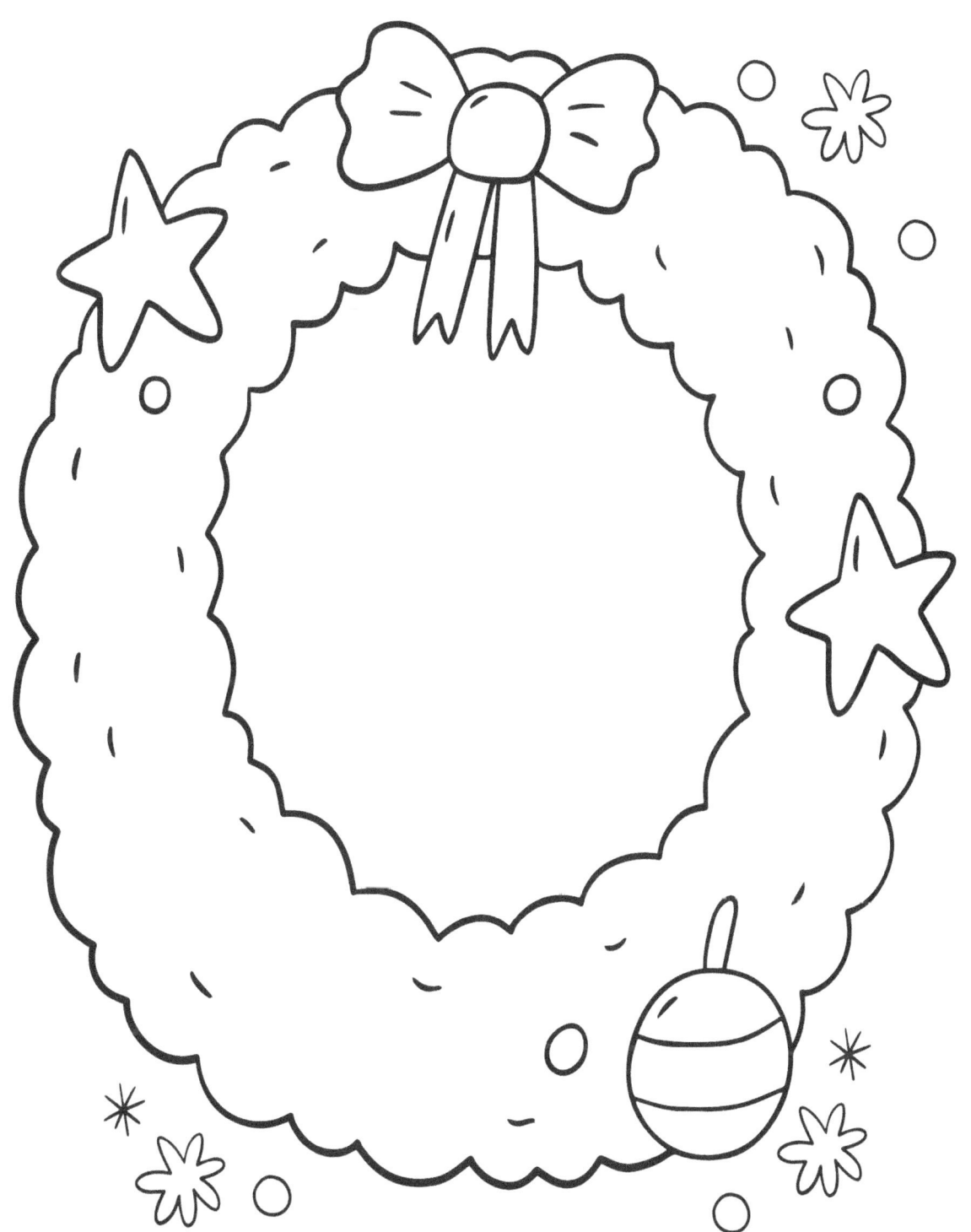

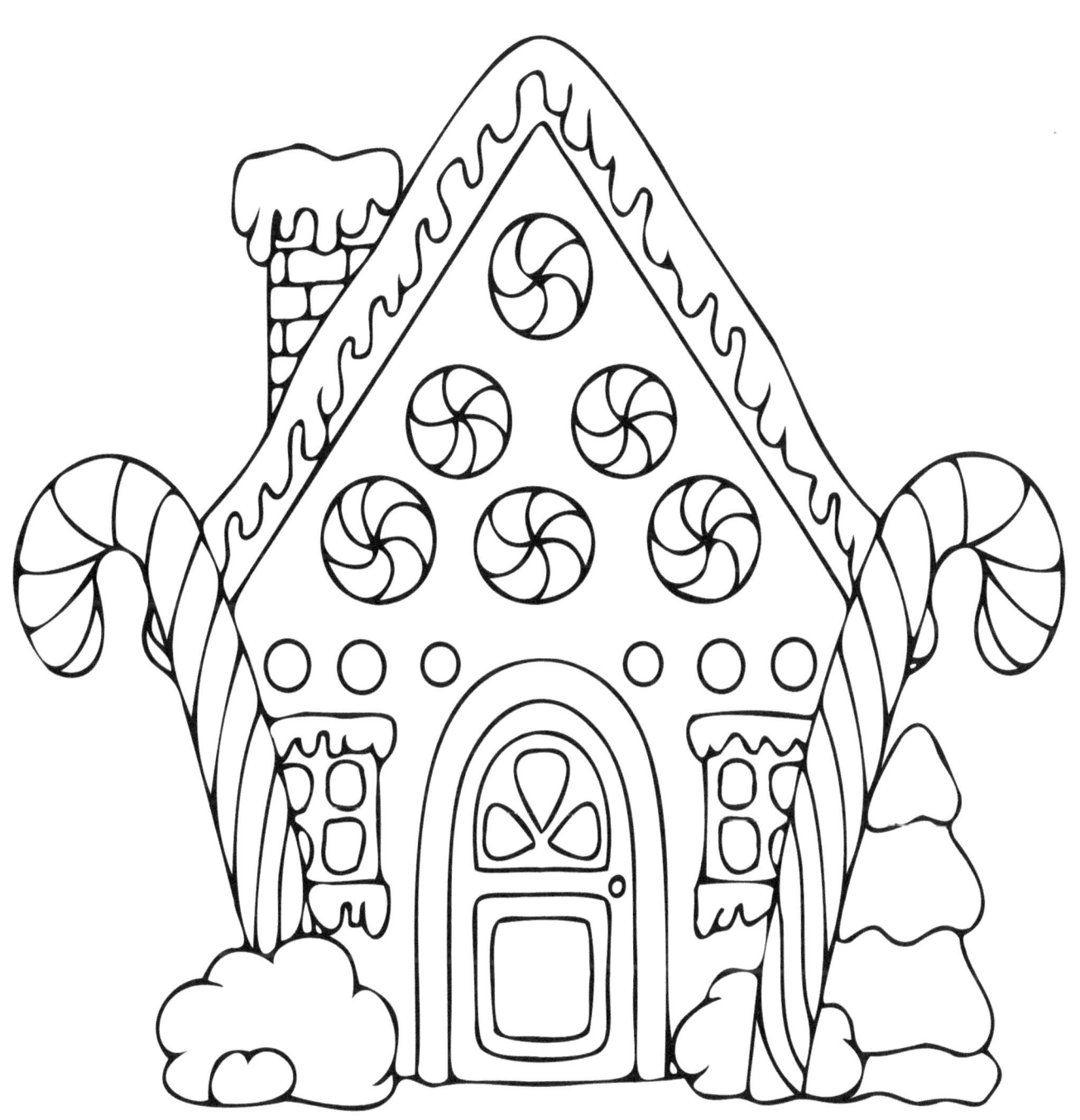

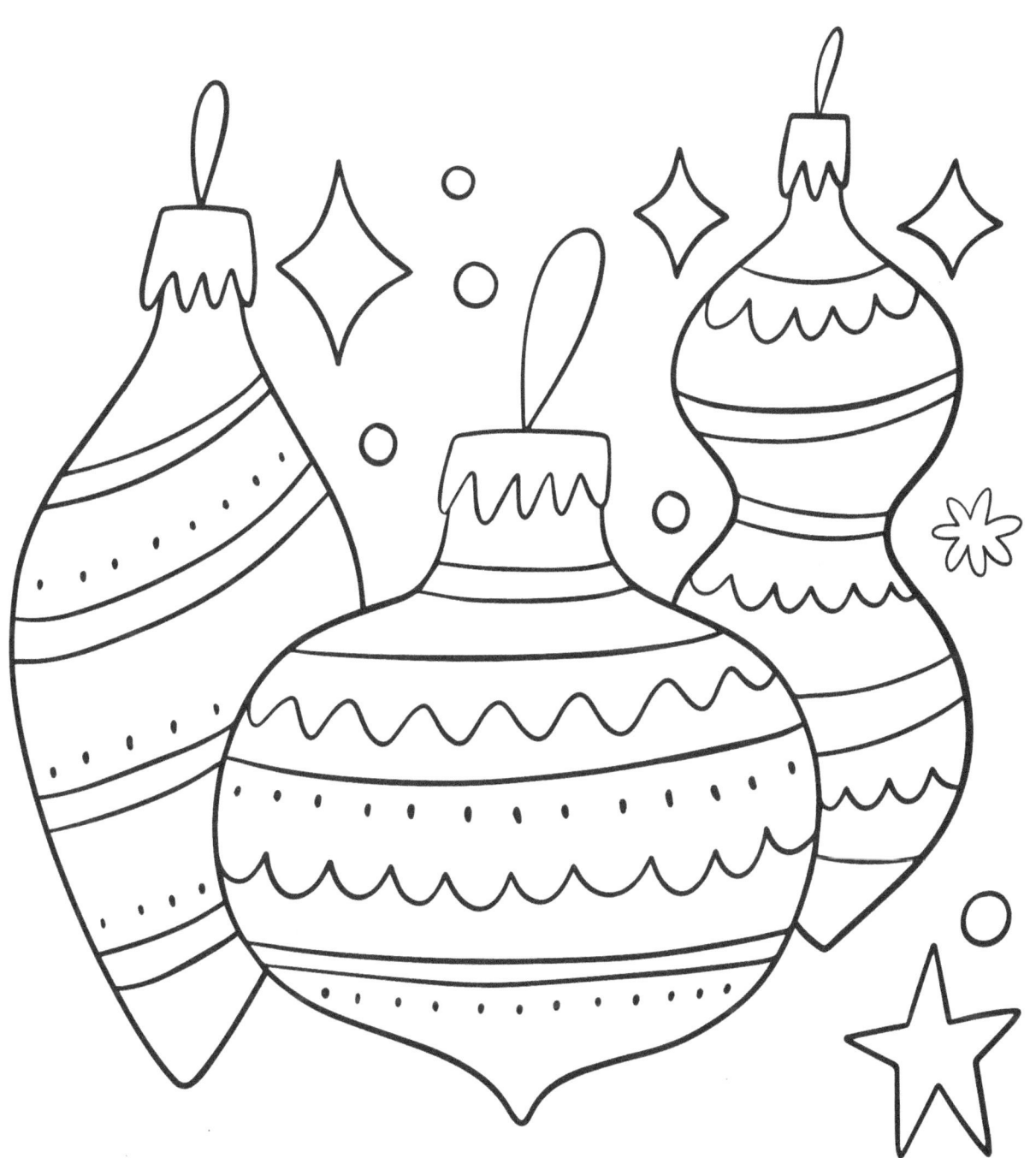

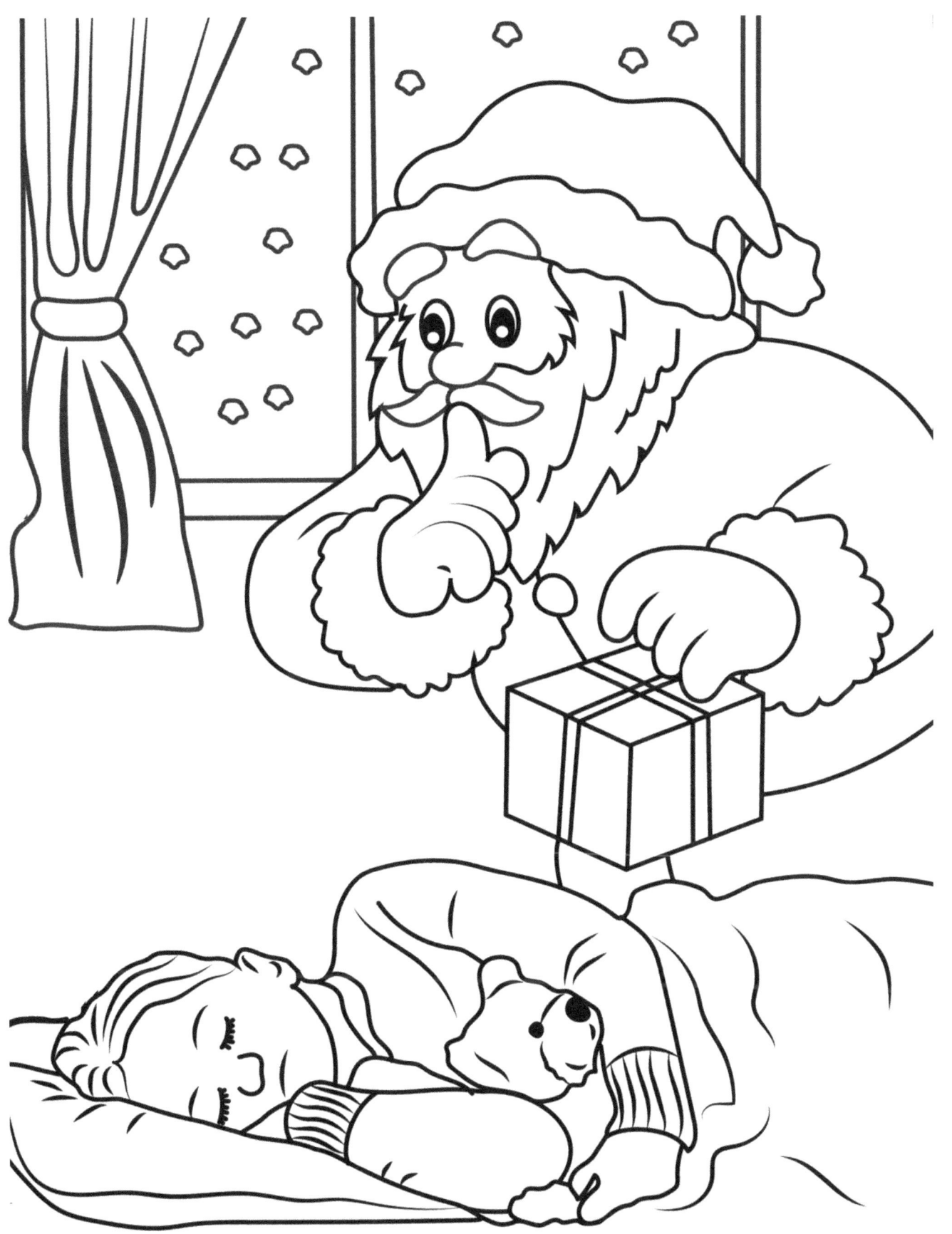

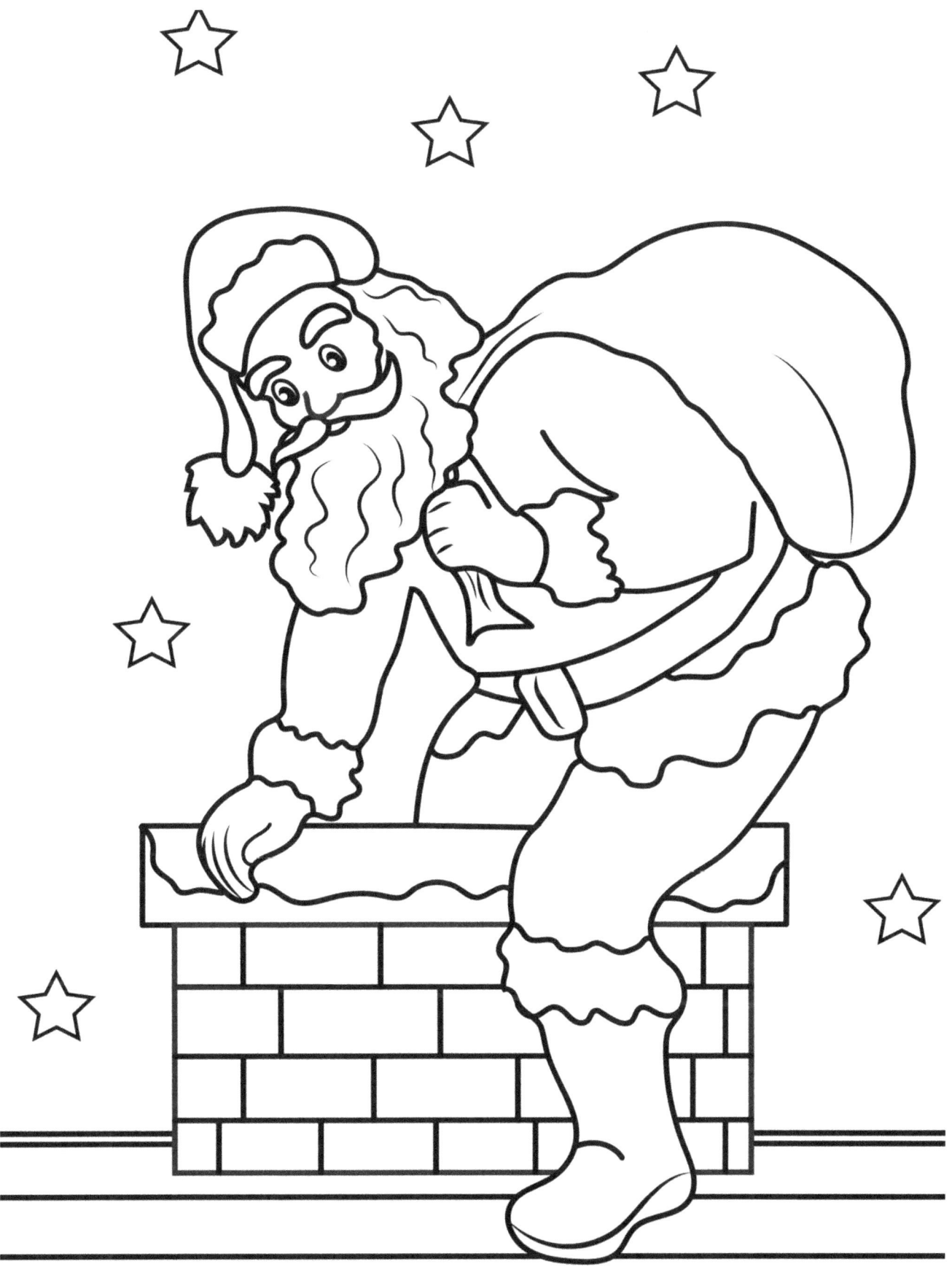

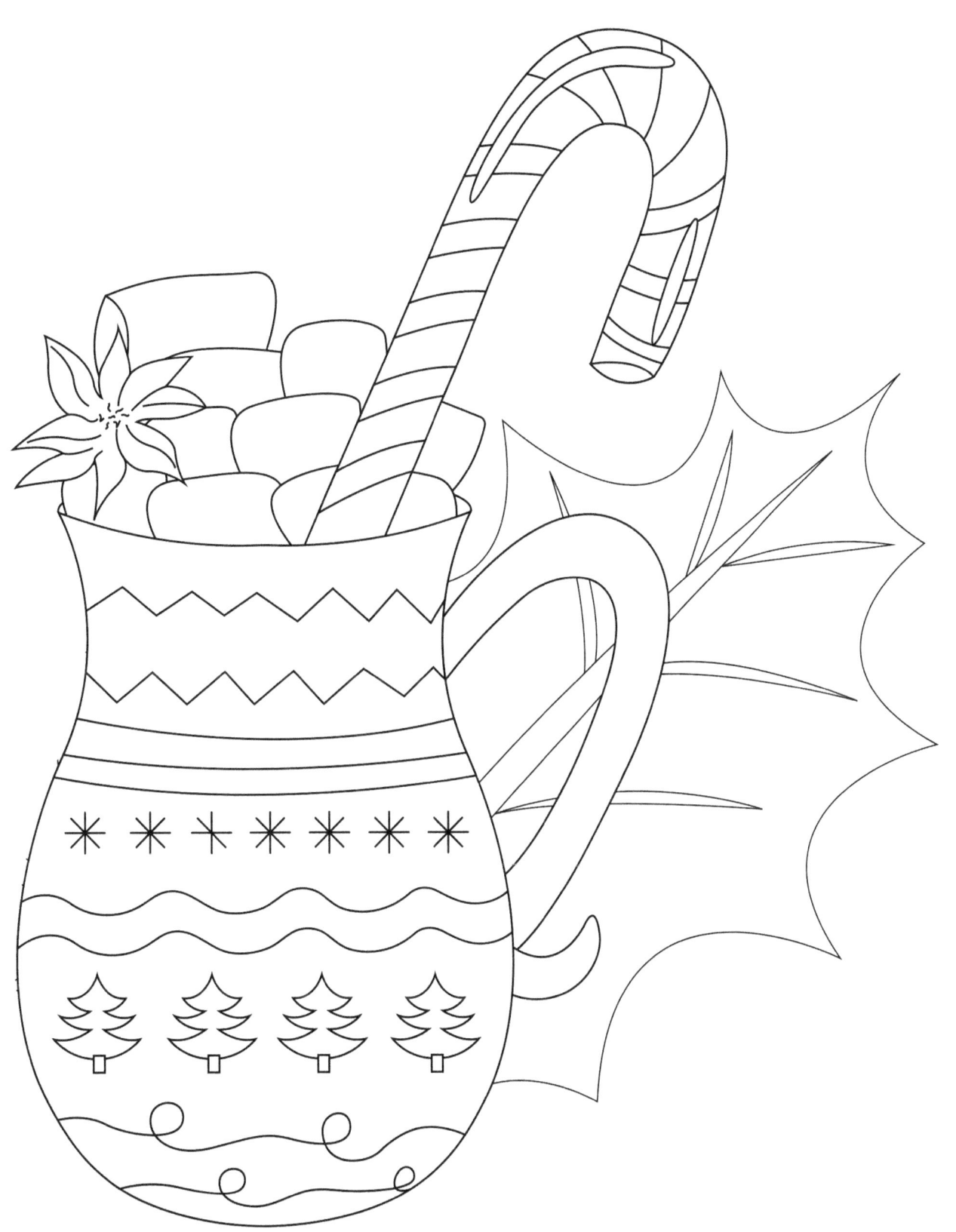

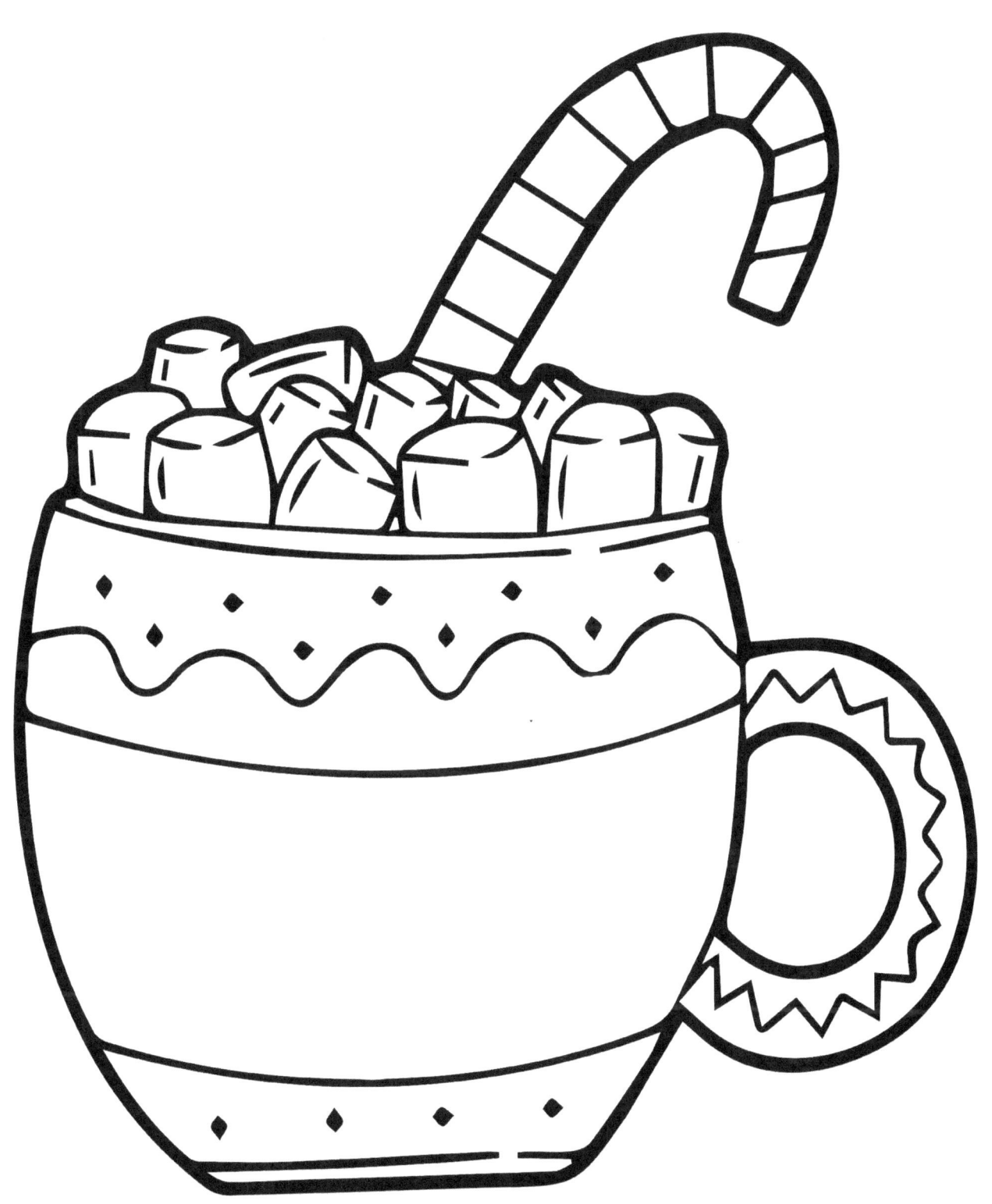

More Books By NEVADA THORNTON:

(Available online at AMAZON or can be ordered from bookstores)

Coloring books for adults relaxation

JOY

NEVADA THORNTON

NEVADA THORNTON
RELAXING
Coloring books for adults relaxation

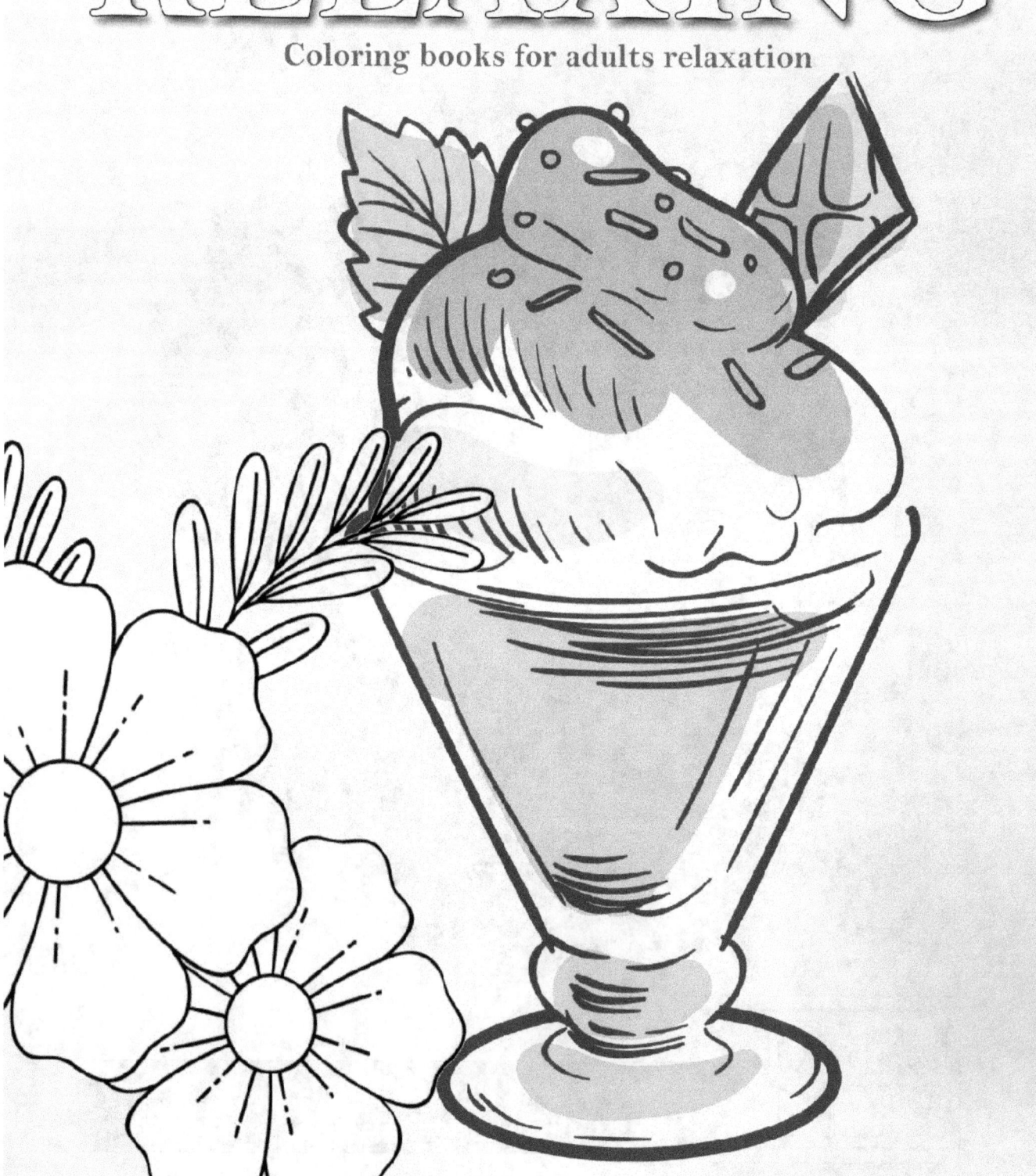

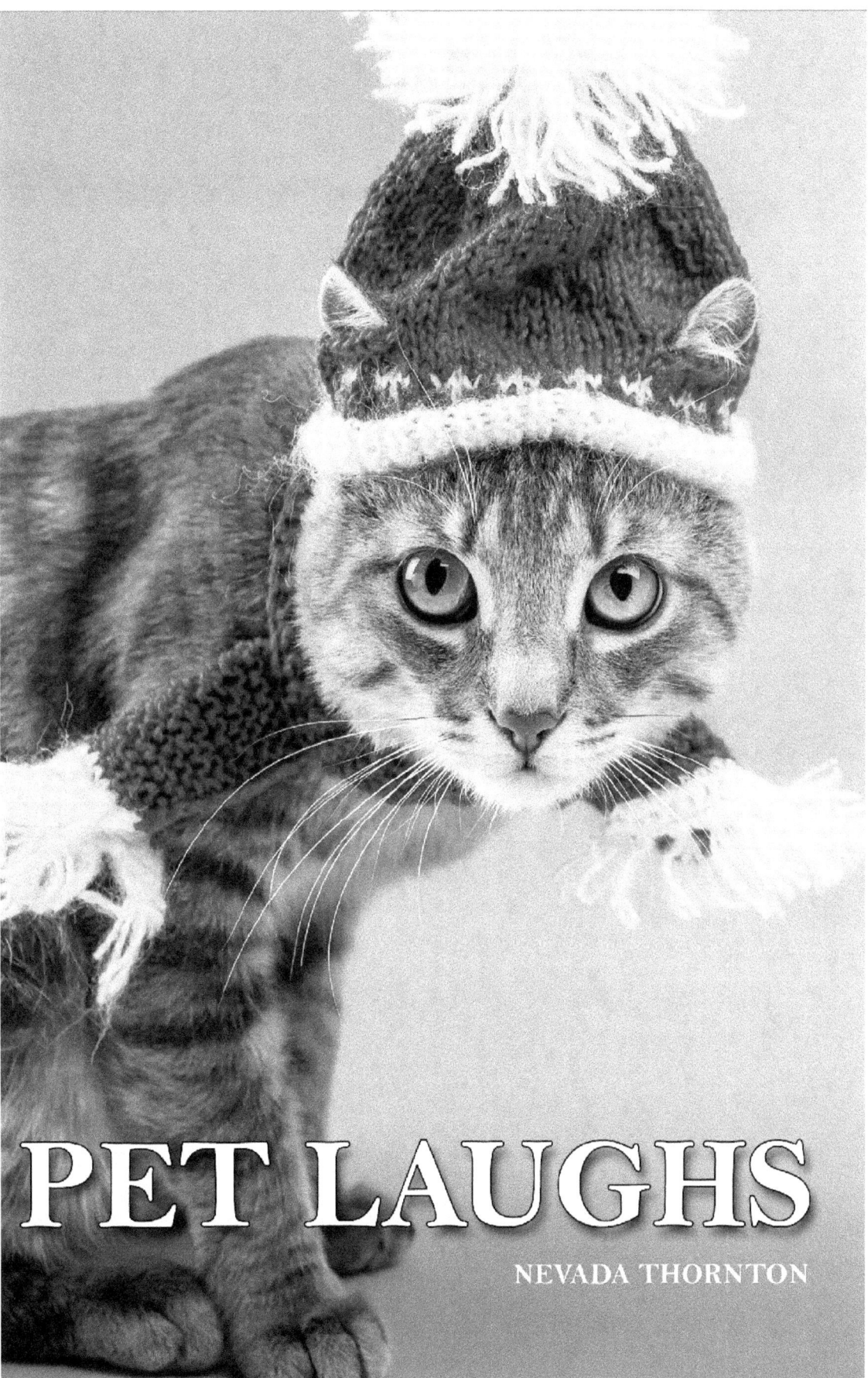

PET LAUGHS

NEVADA THORNTON